NOURISH YOUR SKIN . . .
NOURISH YOURSELF

Includes chapters on . . .

- ◊ THE NEW SUNSCREENS
- ◊ YOUTH-ENHANCING MOISTURIZERS
- ◊ RETINOIDS
- ◊ HYDROXY ACIDS
- ◊ ANTIOXIDANTS
- ◊ BOTANICALS
- ◊ SKIN SECRETS FROM THE SEA
- ◊ CHEMICAL PEELS
- ◊ WRINKLE FILLERS
- ◊ SKIN RESURFACING
- ◊ FACE-LIFTS
- ◊ WRINKLE-REDUCING MAKEUP AND MORE

WRINKLE-FREE
Your Guide to Youthful Skin at Any Age

WRINKLE-FREE

Your Guide to Youthful Skin at Any Age

Maggie Greenwood-Robinson, Ph.D.

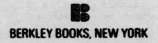

BERKLEY BOOKS, NEW YORK

NOTE: Every effort has been made to ensure that the information contained in this book is complete and accurate. However, neither the publisher nor the author is engaged in rendering professional advice or services to the individual reader. The ideas, procedures, and suggestions contained in this book are not intended as a substitute for consulting with your physician. All matters regarding your health require medical supervision. Neither the author nor the publisher shall be liable or responsible for any loss, injury, or damage allegedly arising from any information or suggestion in this book. The opinions expressed in this book represent the personal views of the author and not of the publisher.

WRINKLE-FREE

A Berkley Book / published by arrangement with the author

PRINTING HISTORY
Berkley edition / September 2001

Copyright © 2001 by Maggie Greenwood-Robinson
Book design by Kristin del Rosario
Cover design by Erika Fusari

All rights reserved.
This book, or parts thereof, may not be reproduced in any form without permission. For information address: The Berkley Publishing Group, a division of Penguin Putnam Inc., 375 Hudson Street, New York, New York 10014.

Visit our website at
www.penguinputnam.com

ISBN: 0-425-18154-5

BERKLEY®
Berkley Books are published by The Berkley Publishing Group, a division of Penguin Putnam Inc., 375 Hudson Street, New York, New York 10014. BERKLEY and the "B" design are trademarks belonging to Penguin Putnam Inc.

PRINTED IN THE UNITED STATES OF AMERICA

10 9 8 7 6 5 4 3

To magazine publisher
Robert Kennedy,
who gave me my first opportunity to write books

CONTENTS

ACKNOWLEDGMENTS

I gratefully thank the following people for their work and contributions to this book: my agent, Madeleine Morel, 2M Communications, Ltd.; Christine Zika and the staff at The Berkley Publishing Group; and my husband, Jeff, for love and patience during the research and writing of this book.

PART ONE

Toward Wrinkle-Free Skin

1

Your Amazing Skin

AT age 28, I noticed my first wrinkles—faint yet still perceptible lines, one under my right lower eyelid and the other under my left. Alarmed, I vowed to look as young I could for as long as I could. I started taking my skin very seriously.

I had once read that actresses slathered petroleum jelly on their faces at night to fight wrinkles, and so I followed suit—religiously. I started using skin-care cosmetics that promised to delay wrinkles indefinitely. I constantly inspected my face for signs of their encroachment. In the years that followed, I tried numerous antiwrinkle products and treatments, doing my best to preserve a youthful complexion.

Has the effort been fruitful? I think so. I discovered that the earlier you start taking care of your skin, the better you'll look at midlife. But even if you begin at 40, 50, 60, or later, you can still restore much of your skin's former glory.

Here's why: Today, more than at any other time in history, there is an amazing array of medically proven products and methods to prevent wrinkles and forestall their progression. And that's exciting, especially for the 76 million baby boomers in America who are entering a new phase of life—aging.

Another question: Is the wrinkle-fighting effort—and in many cases, its associated costs—worth it? I believe so, particularly when you ponder not just the physical satisfaction of looking younger, but also its social and psychological ramifications.

Consider, then, some fascinating research, showing that that attractive, youthful-looking people are:

◊ Perceived by others as having a good personality.

◊ Judged as being warmer, sensitive, and kinder.

◊ Apt to have a happier marriage.

◊ Less depressed, with a more positive outlook on life.

◊ More satisfied with life, in general.

◊ Healthier and likely to live longer than average.

So you see, our looks, especially the way our faces look, can have a powerful impact on our lives. It stands to reason that we'd want to mount a strong defense against wrinkles and other signs of aging.

To learn what can be done to fight wrinkles, it helps to understand some basic skin anatomy. So let's get started on a short biology lesson.

SKIN ANATOMY 101

The skin is the largest and most visible organ of your body, covering approximately two square yards if you stretched it out like a tablecloth. If put on a scale, your skin would weigh about six pounds.

Throughout life, skin performs various vital duties. It protects your body against heat, light, injury, and infection. It also helps regulate your body temperature by making pores larger or smaller; disposes of body wastes; stores water, fat, and vitamin D (which is manufactured in the skin); and contains nerve endings that help you sense pain and pleasure.

Anatomically, your skin is composed of three major layers: the *epidermis,* the *dermis,* and the *subcutaneous fat layer.* These layers are made up of roughly 100 billion cells of various types.

The Epidermis

The epidermis itself is multilayered. When viewed microscopically, it resembles a "brick wall" of cells, with layers of lipids between them. The primary duty of the epidermis is protection against the environment, including light, heat, water loss, toxins, and infectious organisms.

The deepest layer of the epidermis is the *stratum basale.* It contains dividing cells that are transformed into skin cells called *keratinocytes.* Keratinocytes produce keratin, a tough but elastic protein that helps protect the skin from harmful substances. Keratin is also the major structural protein of hair and nails. Approximately 90 percent of all skin cells in the epidermis are keratinocytes.

In a process called *keratinization,* keratinocytes migrate upward through the skin, changing their shape along the way. After they reach their destination—the skin's outer layer—they are eventually sloughed off.

The next layer is the *stratum spinosum,* or "prickly layer," so named for its polygon-shaped keratinocytes that have a prickly appearance. Both the stratum basale and the stratum spinosum contain *melanocytes,* cells that produce granules of *melanin.* Melanin is a natural pigment that gives your skin its characteristic color. By absorbing light energy, melanin protects your skin from excessive ultraviolet radiation. In fact, it darkens with repeated exposure to ultraviolet light—a reaction that produces a suntan.

Melanocytes account for about 2 to 3 percent of all skin cells in the epidermis. The melanin granules they produce are carried to the skin's surface along with the keratinocytes and are eventually shed as well. With age, the number of melanocytes diminishes, resulting in less shielding from ultraviolet light.

Another type of cell found mostly in the stratum spinosum is the *Langerhans cell,* which makes up about 5 percent of the cells residing in the epidermis. Langerhans cells play an important role in immunity, your body's defense against disease. In skin that has been sun-damaged, the number of Langerhans cells in the epidermis falls off by as much as 50 percent. Some medical experts believe that this decline may increase your vulnerability to skin cancer.

Next is the *stratum granulosum.* Keratinocytes in this layer are filled with granules of a substance called *keratohyalin.* Keratohyalin is building blocks of keratin.

Once keratinocytes have made their way to the surface of the skin—a journey that takes an average of 26 to 42 days—they become smaller and flatter. After about two weeks, they eventually die off. The flattened dead keratinocytes are then called *corneocytes,* and they form the visible outer layer of the epidermis, the *stratum corneum.* Though very thin, the stratum corneum is quite tough and resilient. Its corneocytes flake off with washing and friction. Thus, in an ongoing process of renewal, the epidermis is constantly casting off old cells and replacing itself.

The Dermis

The dermis, situated below the epidermis, makes up the bulk of your skin—about 90 percent—and is responsible for its structure and support. The dermis is composed of two layers. Uppermost is the *papillary dermis,* whose surface area contains small, fingerlike projections called *papillae.* The papillae anchor the dermis to the epidermis.

The papillary dermis is reinforced with yellow, rubbery fibers called *elastin,* and tough, white fibers known as *collagen.* Elastin gives your skin elasticity, and collagen provides strength and resiliency.

Collagen is the most abundant protein in the body and makes up about 6 percent of your weight. It composes about 70 percent of the dry weight of the dermis. In addition to creating a supportive structure for skin and other soft tissues, collagen forms scar tissue that heals wounds, the structures that mend bone fractures, and a material in blood vessels that prevents bruising.

Elastin is a rubbery, meshlike protein that makes up about 2 percent of the dry weight of the dermis. You can think of elastin like spandex fabric, with the ability to stretch, then snap back to its original shape. Besides the skin, elastin is found in the ligaments, vocal cords, respiratory organs, large arteries, and spine, among other places.

The papillary dermis also contains a network of blood vessels that nourish the skin and guard against heat loss; lymph vessels that form part of the body's drainage system; and nerve endings that are receptive to touch, pressure, pain, and temperature.

The papillary dermis is permeated with proteins called *glycosaminoglycans* (GAGs) that can hold up to 1,000 times their weight in water. This ability helps moisturize your skin. In addition, GAGs help protect the integrity of collagen by preserving its resilience. The abundance of GAGs in newborn baby's skin makes it smooth and supple. GAGs, however, decline with age.

Beneath the papillary dermis is the *reticular layer,* which also contains collagen, elastin, and blood vessels. Interspersed among these components are specialized structures such as sweat glands, hair follicles, and oil glands (sebaceous glands). The sebaceous glands manufacture a yellowish, oily secretion called *sebum* that can absorb and lock in large amounts of moisture. Sebum is a mixture of fats, cholesterol, proteins, and salts. It protects and lubricates your skin.

Found in the dermis are *fibroblasts,* mother cells that give birth to new collagen and elastin. As you get older, the population of fibroblasts in the skin declines. By the time you're 80, you'll have half the fibroblasts in your dermis as you had at birth.

The Subcutaneous Fat Layer

Under the dermis is the *subcutaneous fat layer,* which insulates your body and serves as a shock absorber. This layer also contains a network of blood vessels, lymph vessels, and nerves. Fat cells, collagen, and elastin reside in the subcutaneous fat layer, too. This layer anchors the reticular layer to your muscles and bones.

TO SUM UP

If biology isn't your thing, don't worry. The point is: Your skin is a versatile, dynamic organ that, unlike other organs, has the power to regenerate itself. But despite its amazing regenerative abilities, there are more than 50 factors at work that age your skin. In the next chapter, we'll explore some of these factors and gain important insights into how they can be controlled.

2

How Your Face Ages

E VERY time you laugh, smile, frown, cry, pucker your lips, raise your eyebrows, or squint your eyes, the muscles of your face contract, temporarily folding your skin into creases. In your youth, when skin is firm, supple, and elastic, these lines of expression vanish immediately as your muscles relax and your skin springs back to smoothness.

But with age, years of sun exposure, and other skin ravagers, your skin loses its youthful bounce. No longer can it retract with its earlier pliability. It begins the process of acquiring, over time, permanent lines—"wrinkles"—on those areas of the face most subjected to muscular contractions. "Crow's-feet" fan out from the corner of the eyes, "marionette" lines run parallel to your nose, and frown lines become etched into your forehead and between your brows.

Call them what you will, these are among the signifiers of aging, or what scientists dispassionately describe as "the progressive loss of tissue structure and function."

What, then, causes this downhill slide?

Aging, in general, is a cumulative series of events, often occurring simultaneously but at different speeds in different individuals. When discussing skin aging, scientists and dermatologists (skin doctors) categorize these events into two broad groups: *intrinsic aging,* the normal skin changes that occur with the passage of time; and *extrinsic aging,* those undesirable skin changes that result from exposure to the environment, as well as from poor lifestyle choices.

INTRINSIC SKIN AGING

During the normal aging process, individual skin cells in the epidermis enlarge and lose their ability to stick together. This process can be compared to a brick wall that is gradually coming apart. The bricks are the epidermal cells, and the mortar is a protein cement that attaches them together. With age, this "mortar" crumbles—a degenerative change that is partly responsible for the dry, scaly skin seen in older adults.

As your skin matures, the renewal rate at which the epidermis sheds and replaces its topmost layer of cells begins to slow down. Between age 30 and 80, your epidermis will gradually thin out.

Your dermis becomes thinner, too. The number of fibroblasts declines, and less collagen is produced. Consequently, the supportive scaffolding provided by the collagen network virtually collapses.

By the time you're 30, elastin fibers have begun to fray like a worn rope and practically disappear by age 70. Your skin loses its original strength and elasticity and, when pressed, is unable to spring back to its original form. The fine wrinkles you notice on your face are a result of these changes.

The loss of elasticity also causes your facial skin to loosen and sag. Aggravating this condition are changes taking place in your facial structure, including a progressive loss of bone in the lower third of your face. Your entire skull thins out, too, causing your skin to sag. Fat cells in the subcutaneous fat layer wither away as well. This hollows out your cheeks and temples, and your face looks gaunt. In essence, there is less bone and fat to prop up your skin, and it takes on a drooping appearance.

What's more, soft tissue in your face begins to redistribute itself, resulting in a more pointy chin and nose. The forces of gravity are at work, too, pulling your skin downward.

As you get older, sweat and oil glands shrink considerably, depriving your skin of its natural moisture and lubrication. Your skin begins to dry out as a result of these changes. You may look paler, too, because aging skin has fewer blood vessels in the papillary dermis.

These changes often occur in cycles over time. They don't happen overnight, of course, but represent a gradual buildup and interplay of specific aging factors. These are discussed below.

Heredity

How well you weather the forces of intrinsic aging depends, to a large degree, on your genes—the basic units of heredity that carry instructions for individual characteristics. For instance, if either or one of your parents had young-looking skin well into their golden years, you may have inherited their genetic fountain of youth.

Scientists now speculate that genetic factors account for anywhere from 25 to 30 percent of the aging process, while our interaction with the environment (extrinsic aging) is responsible for some of the rest. Let's say, for example, that you've inherited good skin genes from your parents, but you've been a sun-worshiper all your life. Your skin may have become prematurely aged as a result of lifelong sun exposure. In other words, how you live impacts how well you age. We all have the power to influence our genetic fate positively or negatively by how we treat our bodies.

Cellular Aging

Skin cells are among those in the body that divide and replicate themselves. Yet, under normal circumstances, they continue to do this only for so long—anywhere from 50 to 60 times—after which they lose their function. This predestined and eventual loss of division capability is technically termed *cellular senescence* and is considered a leading theory of aging.

Derived from the French word *senex* meaning "old," cellular senescence refers to how cells, like our own bodies, age. Cellular senescence is genetically orchestrated and occurs naturally with age. By contrast, the opposite of cellular senescence—uncontrolled cell division—is what leads to cancer.

Scientists have discovered that senescent cells reside in and build up in aging human skin. This accumulation of senescent cells compromises the integrity of skin. Here's why: Before becoming senescent, fibroblasts in the dermis secrete minute amounts of enzymes that degrade collagen and large amounts of enzymes that protect collagen. Collagen thus retains its strength.

But as cells become senescent, the tables turn. Fibroblasts churn out more collagen-degrading enzymes that chew up collagen and produce fewer collagen-protective enzymes. Collagen begins to break down. The net effect is fine wrinkling.

Declining Hormones

Produced by glands, tissues, and organs, hormones are chemical messengers that control various conditions in the body. They travel through the bloodstream, looking for cells fitted with *receptors*. Receptors are like doorbells, signaling the cell to open up and let the hormone in.

Recent scientific evidence suggests that certain skin changes attributed to intrinsic aging, namely thinning of the skin and decreased sebum production, are a result of declining hormone levels, such as estrogen in women and testosterone in men.

In the first 10 years after menopause, collagen declines by about 30 percent—the result of reduced estrogen production. As a result, skin begins to lose its elasticity and thickness.

With declining hormones, the turnover rate of cells falls off, too. In a young face, that rate is about 30 days, but slows to 60 days at age 40 and continues to poke along thereafter.

Many skin specialists, however, believe that estrogen loss is a negligible factor in skin aging. Others feel strongly that hormone replacement therapy (HRT) slows the process of wrinkling. For more information on HRT, see chapter 15.

EXTRINSIC AGING

More damaging to your skin than even the normal consequences of aging is exposure to the environment, otherwise known as extrinsic aging. Environmental offenders that hasten skin aging include chronic sun exposure, heat exposure, smoking, sleep position, and stress. These factors—and the unwanted skin changes they trigger—are discussed at length below.

To see the differences between intrinsic aging and extrinsic aging, simply compare unexposed skin (such as that on your buttocks or breasts) with the skin on your face or arms. Quite probably, your unexposed skin is smooth and baby-soft, because it has rarely seen the light of day!

Table 2.1 lists the symptoms of extrinsic aging and intrinsic aging.

Table 2.1: Differences Between Intrinsic Aging and Extrinsic Aging

INTRINSIC AGING	EXTRINSIC AGING
Thinning of the skin	Coarse, deeper facial wrinkles
Fine facial wrinkles	Freckles
Sagging	Age spots
Loss of skin elasticity	Leathery skin texture
Gaunt facial appearance	Sallow, yellowish, or grayish skin
Pallor	
Dry skin due to the reduction in number of sweat and oil glands	Dry skin due to the reduction in number of sweat and oil glands

Photoaging

Skin's public enemy number one is ultraviolet (UV) radiation from the sun or tanning beds. There are two major types of rays: ultraviolet-A (UVA) and ultraviolet-B (UVB). Both can ravage your skin. The damage they inflict is technically known as "photoaging" or "photodamage."

UVA rays, which are present all year round, generate cellular terrorists called *free radicals*. Chemically, a free radical is a molecule that is missing a part of itself—one of its two orbiting electrons. To regain stability, the free radical seizes an electron from other molecules or ditches its unpaired one. In the process, the free radical wreaks molecular havoc by boring through cell walls and making it easy for bacteria, viruses, and other disease-causing agents to slip in and do often-irreparable harm to tissues. Free-radical damage has been implicated in aging, as well as in diseases such as cancer, heart disease, and cataracts.

UVB rays are present mostly in summertime sun, usually around noon. They scramble DNA—our genetic management system—inside skin cells and undermine the body's ability to repair cells. Researchers who study aging believe that DNA damage accumulates, leading to malfunctioning genes and cells, and with time, deteriorating tissues and organs (including skin). UVB rays can also interfere with our natural protection against free radicals.

Fortunately, though, free radicals aren't allowed to go unchecked. They're squelched by *antioxidants,* which include vitamins C, E, beta-carotene, and certain minerals and enzymes. These heroes simply donate an electron to a free radical but without changing into a radical itself. This action "neutralizes," or stops the dangerous multiplication of still more free radicals.

Normally, free radicals don't cause much of a problem. But when free radicals start outnumbering antioxidants, there's trouble—a condition scientists call *oxidative stress* that leads to aging and disease. With sun-induced oxidative stress, free radicals break down collagen and degenerate elastin fibers until they become a shapeless mass. Skin becomes looser and less elastic, and wrinkling more obvious. In addition, sun exposure promotes skin inflammation, which also creates free radicals.

With photoaging, wrinkles are deeper, with more creases and folds than are seen in the fine wrinkling of intrinsic aging. If photoaging continues, collagen production in the dermis falls off at the rate of about 1 percent a year.

Changes occur in skin cells, too. Keratinocytes are damaged. Melanocytes are gradually killed off, whereas in normal aging, they decline. The freckles you see on your skin as you get older are actually dead melanocytes.

Depending on how advanced the photoaging, facial wrinkles may be visible only when you speak, smile, frown, or otherwise show emotion. With more serious photoaging, wrinkles are obvious even when your face is at rest.

Skin color gradually changes from a normal pink glow to a yellowish, sallow tinge. This is caused by the accumulation of degenerated collagen and elastin in the papillary dermis.

Skin also loses its smoothness and turns leathery. This leathery appearance is caused mostly by abnormal deposits of GAGs in the skin. With photoaging, GAGs increase, and are distributed among degenerated elastin fibers rather than in the papillary dermis where they normally belong. Some researchers speculate that the misplacement of GAGs makes them unavailable as a source of natural moisture for the skin. The surface texture of the skin becomes rough and wrinkled as a result. There is also a drop in sebum production with photoaging, causing dry skin.

The areas of the body most affected by photoaging are the face, the back of the neck, neckline, arms, and hands. Skin begins to look old before its time.

People most susceptible to photoaging and wrinkling are those who spend a lot of time in the sun: lifeguards, sunbathers, outdoor athletes, construction workers, farmers, fishermen, among others. If you're fair-skinned, have red or blond hair, or green or gray eyes, signs of photoaging may make their mark as early as your twenties. Darker-skinned individuals, however, are less prone to photoaging. African-Americans, for example, have fewer wrinkles and less facial sagging than do Caucasians, probably because there is more sun-blocking melanin in their epidermis. Regardless, chronic sun exposure can take its toll, no matter what your ethnic heritage.

Heat Damage

Radiant heat from stoves, furnaces, fire, and other such sources can cause skin changes similar to those found in chronically sun-damaged skin. Skin researchers have seen proof of this in bakers and kitchen workers exposed to direct heat from stovetops and ovens for many years. The skin on their faces and arms often ages prematurely. Similar signs of aging have been observed in the skin of people who habitually use space heaters, woodburning stoves, and fireplaces.

Smoking

Crisscrossing facial lines, deeply grooved crow's-feet, vertical furrows above the upper lip, and grayish skin—these are the unsightly characteristics of a "smoker's face." The nicotine in tobacco constricts the blood vessels that carry nutrients to the skin, resulting in prominent wrinkles and prematurely aged skin. In fact, some 40-year-old heavy smokers have the crow's-feet of 60-year-old nonsmokers and are nearly five times more likely to have excessive wrinkles, according to one study.

Skin specialists believe that smoking suffocates the skin by robbing it of oxygen. In fact, studies show that while you smoke, there is a 30 percent decrease in oxygen to the skin. Further, smoking deposits nicotine and its by-products into the tiny blood vessels feeding the skin.

Also, smoking activates collagen-degrading enzymes and produces free radicals. These actions accelerate the breakdown of collagen and elastin in the dermis and pave the way for wrinkles.

Sleep Position

The position in which you sleep has a rather significant effect on facial wrinkling—a fact that was discovered during sleep studies conducted in the early eighties and confirmed recently with new research. It is now known that if you sleep eight hours or more with your face pressed against the pillow or bed, creases will develop on your face. These wrinkles tend to form across the forehead, down the side of the nose, under the eyes as a horizontal line, or as a long vertical line down the cheek. However, these lines are less likely to develop, or be permanent, if you routinely sleep on your back.

Stress

Though not well researched, the effects of unresolved stress on skin aging are fairly obvious. Case in point: Compare the faces of U.S. presidents at the onset of their terms with their faces after they leave office. In a nutshell, they've aged drastically. It is only logical to assume that stress plays a huge role.

Stress does assault your immune system, right down to the cellular level. Recently, scientists discovered that Langerhans cells—immune-system cells found in the skin and other tissues—can communicate with nerve cells through special receptors.

"Therefore, it is reasonable to conclude that the immune system may be influenced by thoughts and other functions of the brain," write Reverend Michael R. Bilkis, M.D., and Kenneth A. Mark, M.D., in *Archives of Dermatology*. "If this is so, then we can also conclude that most of the common dermatologic problems such as adult acne, rosacea, eczema, psoriasis, and other nonspecific inflammatory disorders may be directly influenced by the patient's thoughts and emotions."

Thus, it appears that many common skin disorders are caused or aggravated by chronic stress. These detract from your appearance and may cause skin to stay in a chronic state of inflammation. Inflammation increases free-radical activity, which ages the skin.

Other Factors

In addition to those mentioned above, other environmental factors may speed up skin aging. These include pollution, particularly ozone, which produces free radicals that damage cells, leading to wrinkles.

Yo-yo dieting—the practice of going on and off diets and up and down in weight—can cause wrinkles, too. When you gain weight, skin stretches to compensate. But with a quick, drastic loss in weight, skin can't shrink and retract fast enough, so it sags. You look older and more wrinkled.

BECOMING WRINKLE-FREE

Preventing, minimizing, or erasing wrinkles may sound like an impossible task, but happily, there's plenty you can do to save and restore your skin—even if you've let your skin-care program slide in the past. The standard good skin advice—limiting sun exposure, eating a diet high in fruits and vegetables, drinking lots of water, and quitting smoking—still stands. But today, researchers, dermatologists, and plastic surgeons have products, treatments, and procedures that can help iron out wrinkles and rejuvenate your skin. All of these strategies are covered in this book.

So—let's find out what really works, and how to turn back the facial aging clock, once and for all.

PART TWO

Wrinkle Stoppers

3
First Things First:
The New Sunscreens

THE best defense against wrinkles is not one of the newest or more glamorous treatments on the market. It's one of the oldest—sunscreen—a skin-saving product that has been with us since the twenties. Ironically, though, in that same decade, renowned French designer Coco Chanel popularized the bronzed, tanned look when she employed tanned models to display her fashions. And voilà, the myth of the healthy tan as a symbol of beauty, athleticism, and fitness was born.

But as dermatologist Karen E. Burke, M.D., Ph.D., wrote in the medical journal *Postgraduate Medicine:* "There is no such thing as a healthy tan. A tan is actually the visible evidence of damage to the skin—the very same damage that causes 90 percent of the appearance of aging as well as skin cancer."

Such advice goes largely ignored, however. So does the advice to wear sunscreen. Some proof: A poll of women living in Florida found that 75 percent of the respondents felt that having a tan made them look healthy and attractive. In another poll, college students said that they looked better with a tan; that a suntanned skin is more attractive; and that suntans look healthy. Further, survey after survey reveals that on average, only half of the people on a beach on any given day wear sunscreen.

Still, dermatologists will tell you that slathering on a sunscreen before you go outdoors is the most important antiwrinkle step you can take. If you had begun using sunscreen as a child, chances are you wouldn't have many wrinkles today. But not to worry. If your skin is showing the ugly signs of sun damage, there's still time to make up for lost time. Skin is very forgiving and will repair itself if given the proper care.

SOLAR SAVVY

Topically applied sunscreens defend your skin against the harmful ultraviolet rays of the sun. Over time, those rays gradually disintegrate collagen and elastin, causing saggy skin, wrinkles, and premature skin aging. Excessive sun exposure also interferes with the normal process of skin-cell formation. Cells lose their ability to hold water, too, and skin turns dry and dull.

Sunlight stimulates the abnormal production of pigment-forming melanocytes. They start churning out excess melanin, which ends up causing freckles and age spots. To make matters worse, sun exposure batters Langerhans cells in the skin, which are guardians against disease. This assault on your immune system increases your risk of skin cancer, including the deadliest form—malignant melanoma. (One in five Americans today is diagnosed with skin cancer.)

Not all sunlight is the same. Of all the solar rays reaching the earth, about 56 percent is infrared light, and 39 percent is visible light. The rest is ultraviolet (UV) light. Although making up a smaller percentage of solar energy, UV light inflicts the most bodily harm.

Ultraviolet radiation is the strongest between 10 A.M. and 3 P.M. Even on cloudy days, as much as 50 percent of the sun's ultraviolet light still reaches the earth's surface. UV rays go through water, too. When you're immersed under water, 80 percent of the sun's ultraviolet light can penetrate to your skin. What's more, sand, snow, and concrete reflect up to 85 percent of sunlight, and those reflected rays can strike you in the shade.

The intensity of ultraviolet radiation varies, seasonally and geographically. For instance, UV light is most intense during the summer months, at high altitudes, and in areas closest to the equator. Intensity decreases as latitudes increase.

UV light itself is made up of three different wavelengths: UVC, UVB, and UVA. Most UVC rays and a large portion of UVB rays are deflected by the ozone layer, located approximately 5 to 10 miles above sea level. But UVA light is not deflected, and very large amounts hit the earth. In fact, about 10 to 100 times more UVA light reaches the earth than UVB light does. Tanning booths emit mostly UVA light and some UVB light (about 5 percent.)

All three wavelengths affect the skin in different ways. The small amount of UVC light that makes it to earth is soaked up by the topmost layer of the epidermis. It can cause mild skin reddening.

UVB light penetrates the epidermis and is the chief cause of sunburn. In fact, it has been dubbed the "sunburn radiation." UVB light disarms your skin's natural antioxidant defense system, rendering it virtually powerless against skin-damaging free radicals. UVB light also causes skin cancer by damaging cellular DNA and depleting the skin of immune-protective Langerhans cells. UVB rays can be blocked by window glass and by many sunscreens.

UVA light infiltrates both the epidermis and the dermis. In the skin, it generates free radicals. They harm cellular proteins such as collagen and elastin, and damage the lipid structure of cells. The net effect is accelerated and premature skin aging.

There are actually two subcategories of UVA radiation: UVA I and UVA II. Scientists believe that UVA I is the wavelength most responsible for causing wrinkles because it penetrates more deeply into the dermis. Yet very few sunscreens fully protect against UVA I.

Although most sunburn is caused by UVB rays, about 15 to 20 percent of sunburn is a result of exposure to UVA light. Like UVB light, UVA radiation is linked to skin cancer because it also damages DNA and your immune system. Window glass does not block UVA rays.

Fortunately, sunscreens can help rescue your skin from the ravages of ultraviolet light. Medical research has found that sunscreen protects immune cells from damage, reduces the incidence of sunburn cells (which indicate DNA damage), and guards against skin aging and skin cancer.

CHOOSING THE RIGHT NUMBER: SUN PROTECTION FACTOR (SPF)

When buying a sunscreen, one bit of important label information to check is its *sun protection factor* or SPF, for short. This term describes how long you can stay out in the sun without sunscreen before getting a sunburn. For example, if you normally burn in 15 minutes without sun protection, using an SPF of 4 means you could stay in the sun 60 minutes before you'd burn. This was calculated by multiplying 4 times 15. Put another way, you can stay in the sun four times longer as you would without protection. Using an SPF of 15 would let you stay in the sun 15 times longer.

SPF ratings range from 2 to 30 and higher. The higher the SPF, the greater your protection against UVB rays, in particular. (The SPF rating refers to UVB blockage only.)

Sunscreens with an SPF of 15 will protect your skin against 93 to 95 percent of UVB radiation.

The FDA has classified sunscreens into three categories of protection, based on SPF:

◊ Minimum protection is an SPF of 2 to 11.

◊ Moderate protection is an SPF of 12 to 29.

◊ High protection is an SPF of 30 or higher.

By law, these designations must appear on the labels of sunscreens.

Most physicians recommend using sunscreens with an SPF of 15. Others believe, however, that sunscreens with an SPF of 30 afford better protection against skin damage. These shield against 97 percent of the UVB radiation. In one medical experiment, researchers found that people protected by an SPF 30 sunscreen had 2.5 times fewer sunburned cells than those using an SPF 15 product. In plain terms, the SPF 30 more than doubled the protection.

Controversy simmers over whether using an SPF higher than 30 is warranted. With higher-SPF sunscreens, the FDA feels that there is a greater risk of allergic reactions from higher levels of chemicals on the skin. Further, the agency argues that higher-SPF sunscreens give people a false sense of security and encourage them to stay out in the sun longer, increasing skin damage and risk of skin cancer. It is important to add that higher-SPF sunscreens are often more expensive.

The amount of sunscreen you rub on your skin affects its SPF. Let's say, for example, you coat yourself with only half as much SPF 15 as is recommended on the label. Guess what? Your actual sun protection now falls to a mere 4! So if you apply sunscreen very thinly or unevenly, you may be getting just a smidgen of what you really need.

So that you won't broil your skin, apply the recommended amount: one ounce (about a shot glass full) over your entire body and one-half to a full teaspoon of sunscreen on your face.

Types of Sunscreens

At present, hundreds of brands of topical sunscreens line the shelves of stores. These products are generally divided into two categories: physical sunscreens—better known as *sunblocks*—and chemical sunscreens.

Sunblocks

Sunblocks sit on top of your skin and are not absorbed. They physically stop all ultraviolet radiation from reaching the skin by reflecting or scattering harmful ultraviolet rays. Topical sunblocks are thick, whitish, opaque creams that are usually visible after application. It is the sunblock's opacity that blocks the sun's rays. Examples of sunblocking ingredients include zinc oxide, titanium dioxide, magnesium silicate, ferric chloride, kaolin, red petroleum, and talc.

Of these agents, the most commonly used are zinc oxide and titanium oxide. Both contain mineral particles that absorb UV light. A key advantage of these ingredients is that they can effectively stop wrinkle-promoting UVA I rays—something most traditional sunscreens don't do. Also, one study found that a sunscreen formulated with these oxides helped prevent DNA damage to skin cells. Neither is irritating to the skin.

Zinc oxide, in particular, is best known as the white sticky cream coating the noses of sunbathers, beachgoers, and lifeguards. Now you can purchase a transparent form of zinc oxide in a product called Z-Cote. It is made up of microfine particles, believed to more effectively absorb

UV rays because of their tiny size. In one study, Z-Cote protected against UVB and UVA radiation.

Chemical Sunscreens

Chemical sunscreens, on the other hand, absorb ultraviolet rays. They contain various chemicals that, when combined, can provide a high SPF. Many sunscreens are formulated with sunblocking agents, too. (See table 3.1 for a list of chemicals used in sunscreens.)

Newer sunscreens provide broad-coverage protection, meaning that they screen out both UVA and UVB rays. A sunscreen agent called Parsol 1789, recently approved by the FDA, can block up to two-thirds of UVA light and protects throughout the UVA spectrum (UVA I and UVA II)— so check your sunscreen for this ingredient.

Well absorbed by the skin, Parsol 1789 is usually combined with UVB blockers for maximum sun protection. In fact, sunscreens containing Parsol and titanium oxide or zinc oxide block at least 80 percent of the sun's UVA rays.

Sunscreens are also available as "water resistant" (will last 40 minutes in the water) and "very water resistant" (will last 80 minutes in the water). These are good choices if you swim or participate in water sports.

Unlike sunblocks, sunscreens are invisible after application. They come as creams, lotions, gels, sprays, and wax sticks. If you have very dry skin, you might opt for a sunscreen in a creamy base. However, these sunscreens can leave an oily film on your skin that attracts sand and airborne particles. Instead, you might opt for a product that dries on contact with your skin.

One of the newest sunscreens on the market is Sunbar from Sunsation Tanning Products. Available in grocery stores and pharmacies, it is a solid soap bar containing sunscreens and sunblocks. You apply it while showering. Sunbar provides an SPF of 15 to 24 and protection against UVA, UVB, and UVC rays.

Table 3.1: Sunscreen Ingredients

ACTIVE INGREDIENTS	BLOCKAGE	IMPORTANT INFORMATION
PABA and PABA esters *PABA* *Padimate O,* *Padimate A* *Glyceryl PABA*	Screens UVB rays.	Pure PABA can irritate the skin; PABA esters are less irritating. PABA is rarely used.
Salicylates *Octyl methoxycin-* *namate (OMC)* *Ethylhexyl* *p-methoxycinnamate* *Octocrylene* *Cinoxate*	Screens UVB rays. OMC also protects against UVA II.	Rarely produces allergic reactions. OMC is found in more than 90 percent of sunscreens; octocrylene is used in many recreational sunscreens. Cinnoxate is rarely used.
Benzophenones *Oxybenzone* *Dioxybenzone* *Sulisobenzone*	Screens UVB and UVA II rays.	Provides broad coverage; may cause skin irritation. Dioxybenzone is rarely used.
Anthranilites *Menthyl anthranilite*	Screens UVA II rays.	Absorbs UVA light.
Parsol 1789 (avobenzone)	Screens UVA I and II rays.	Very effective UVA absorber; rarely causes allergic reactions.
Sunblocks *Zinc oxide* *Titanium dioxide* *Magnesium silicate* *Ferric chloride* *Kaolin* *Red petroleum* *Talc*	Provide UVB and UVA protection.	Rarely causes skin irritation; is visible after application. Most commonly used are zinc oxide and titanium oxide. Both block UVA I and UVA II rays.

Adapted from: Wentzell, J.M. 1996. Sunscreens: the ounce of prevention. *American Family Physician* 53: 1713–1733; Mitchnick, M., et al. 1998. A review of sunscreen safety and efficacy. *Photochemistry and Photobiology* 68: 243–256.

Other Skin-Friendly Ingredients

Many sunscreens are formulated with moisture-providing ingredients that soothe the skin plus protect it from peeling. One of these ingredients is topical vitamin E, which reduces skin damage from UV radiation and acts as a natural moisturizer. (For more information on topical vitamin E, see chapter 7.)

Another widely used ingredient in sunscreens is aloe vera. A member of the lily family, aloe is an African succulent plant. Its leaves are filled with an antibacterial and antifungal gel that appears to be useful as a topical agent for treating wounds and healing burns. The gel also acts as an anti-inflammatory agent and contains a number of helpful chemicals that naturally stimulate the immune system. In addition, aloe contains an antioxidant enzyme called *superoxide dismutase,* which is one of the body's natural defenses against skin-damaging free radicals.

SIDE EFFECTS OF TOPICAL SUNSCREENS

Chemical sunscreens have virtually no side effects, with the exception of eye stinging or occasional mild skin irritation. Fortunately, some sunscreens, such as Neutrogena 15 and Coppertone Sport, are formulated so that they don't stray into the eyes.

Active ingredients such as p-aminobenzoic acid (PABA), preservatives, and other additives can provoke allergic reactions in the skin. Symptoms include redness or tiny pimplelike bumps on the skin. Newer sunscreens containing Parsol usually do not cause such reactions. What's more, PABA esters such as Padimate O, Padimate A, and glyceryl PABA have generally replaced pure PABA in sunscreens because they are less irritating.

There is some concern over whether sunscreen interferes with the body's production of vitamin D, a nutrient
involved in the formation and maintenance of healthy
bones and teeth. Sunlight activates a substance in the skin
called pre–vitamin D_3 and converts it into vitamin D. Some
skin researchers believe that sunscreen decreases or blocks
the synthesis of D_3 in the skin, particularly in the elderly.
With age, there's a natural falloff in the body's ability to
make its own vitamin D anyway, and it's theorized that
sunscreen aggravates this situation. Medical studies
haven't totally verified this, though. Nonetheless, many
physicians and other health-care practitioners recommend
that older people who use sunscreens should eat one or
more servings of dairy products a day or take a daily vitamin D supplement.

GUIDELINES FOR OPTIMUM PROTECTION

If you're really serious about protecting your skin and preventing wrinkles, here are some important guidelines to
follow:

◊ Select higher-SPF sunscreens (at least 15). Use an
   SPF 30 sunscreen if your skin is very sensitive
   and fair, you spend the entire day in the sun, you
   have a lot of moles or a family or personal history
   of skin cancer, or you are taking a drug that increases sensitivity to sun (see below).

◊ Read the label to make sure the sunscreen provides UVB and UVA protection.

◊ Don't be chintzy. Use a liberal portion of sunscreen. It takes about one ounce to fully coat your
   body.

◊ Apply sunscreen at least 30 minutes before going out. That way, it has an opportunity to weld with the topmost layer of the epidermis (the stratum corneum) and will work better.

◊ Opt for water-resistant sunscreens if you swim or play water sports.

◊ Reapply every two hours, particularly after swimming or playing sports. Reapply immediately if the sunscreen has been rubbed off your body.

◊ Use sunscreen even if you're sitting under a beach umbrella. The umbrella will shield you from only 40 to 50 percent of the sun's radiation.

◊ Avoid sunscreens formulated with fragrances or benzocaine. These ingredients can irritate your skin.

◊ Makeup can be applied over your sunscreen. (Many makeup foundations are formulated with sunscreen; if you wear this type of makeup, choose one with an SPF of at least 15.)

◊ Wear UV-protective sunglasses, a wide-brimmed hat, and tight-weave clothing while in the sun. Wearing a baseball cap will keep sun off most of your forehead. Generally, proper clothing provides an SPF of up to 60 for UVB rays, but will protect you across the entire UV spectrum.

◊ Avoid peak times for UVB exposure—from 10 A.M. to 3 P.M.

◊ Avoid tanning beds or sunlamps.

◊ Don't stay out in the sun longer than you would ordinarily just because you've applied sunscreen.

SUNLESS TANNING

If want a tan but not the wrinkles it eventually brings, try using sunless tanning lotions, also called self-tanners. Available as creams, lotions, or sprays, they contain harmless cosmetic dyes such as dihydroxyacetone (DHA). DHA reacts with a protein in the skin to produce a temporary tan. Some tanning products contain a sunscreen.

Sunless tanning products are safe and effective, although they sometimes impart an orangish tinge to the skin. To avoid this, use a product with a low level of DHA. One such product is Lancôme's Flash Bronzer Body Spray with SPF 15.

To ensure an even "tan," exfoliate your skin with a loofah sponge beforehand. Moisturizing your skin before applying the self-tanner will help prevent streaking. Apply the sunless tanning product using a circular motion. Don't use as much on your elbows, ankles, heels, or knees, since these areas tend to soak up too much stain.

Avoid rubbing the product into your hairline, since sunless tanners can stain your hair. After application, wash your hands thoroughly to remove the excess.

A FINAL NOTE:
WHEN SUNLIGHT AND DRUGS DON'T MIX

Attention sunbathers: If you're taking certain medicines, don't go out in the sun for prolonged periods of time or you could run the risk of severe sunburn, hives, swelling or blistering of the skin, premature skin aging, or other serious health problems.

The reason is that many commonly prescribed drugs and over-the-counter medicines can make your skin abnormally sensitive to light. These drugs can make you *photosensitive*.

Drugs that induce photosensitive reactions include antidepressants and tranquilizers; antihistamines, used in cold and allergy medicines; cardiovascular medications for the treatment of high blood pressure; anticancer drugs; antibiotics; anticonvulsants; acne drugs such as Retin-A; diuretics (water pills); diabetes drugs; nonsteroidal anti-inflammatory drugs (NSAIDs), when taken in dosages for the treatment of arthritis; and topical first-aid creams. Even the popular herb Saint-John's-wort, which is taken for depression, can make your skin more sensitive to light. Most photosensitizing drugs carry a warning label.

All of these medications contain chemicals called *photoreactive agents* that bring about changes in the skin after exposure to UV radiation, either from natural sunlight or an artificial source such as a tanning booth. Even light generated from a photocopier has been known to trigger photosensitivity!

Photosensitive reactions fall into two categories: photoallergic and phototoxic. Some drugs produce both types of reactions.

A photoallergic reaction is the result of changes in immunity and is set in motion when UV light structurally alters the drug. The drug then acts as a *hapten,* a substance that binds to proteins in the skin and stimulates antibody production as part of an immune-system response. This leads to an allergic reaction that manifests itself in skin itching, swelling, and redness within seconds after sun exposure. Your skin may develop a pimply rash that resembles poison ivy. Areas of skin not exposed to light may be affected, too.

Drugs capable of causing photoallergies include psychiatric medications; antimicrobial agents; minoxidil, used in the treatment of hair loss; NSAIDs such as ketoprofen prescribed for arthritis; thiazides, a class of diuretics taken for high blood pressure; and benzocaine, for treating middle-ear infections.

Photoallergies can persist, too, even after you stop taking the offending medication. In one study, researchers found several patients who continued to have skin problems for up to 20 years—even after discontinuing the photoreactive medicine and avoiding further use of such drugs. Also, photoallergy can strike again if you come into contact with agents that are chemically similar to the original photosensitizing drug.

A phototoxic reaction, which is more common, looks and feels like a severe sunburn with inflammation, redness, and blisters. It may last 72 hours or more and is very painful. Unlike a photoallergy, a phototoxic reaction does not affect the immune system. Rather, the drug soaks up additional energy UV light and releases that energy into the skin, triggering skin-cell damage. Drugs that can induce phototoxic reactions include psychiatric medications, amiodarone (used to treat heart rhythm disorders), antibiotics such as tetracyline or ofloxacin, and over-the-counter pain relievers such as ibuprofen and naproxen sodium.

Chronic use of photoreactive drugs, combined with long-term sun exposure, can have serious medical consequences. These include premature skin aging, more intense allergic reactions, cataracts, blood-vessel damage, compromised immunity, and skin cancer. In addition, photoreactive drugs can aggravate existing skin problems such as acne, eczema, herpes, or psoriasis.

Treating Photosensitivity

Should symptoms of photosensitivity appear after you've been out in the sun, see your doctor or dermatologist right away. Treatment typically involves the use of oral or topical corticosteroids, a class of powerful drugs that reduce inflammation and suppress photoallergic reactions; antihistamines to stop any itching; and sunscreen to further protect your skin. You may also want to take a cool bath or shower.

In addition, you'll be instructed to limit your time in the sun and drink plenty of liquids to prevent dehydration. To ease symptoms, your doctor may reduce the dosage of the photosensitizing drug, or replace it with one less likely to provoke an adverse reaction. Symptoms usually disappear within a week after you begin protecting your skin from the sun and avoiding the photosensitizing drug.

What You Can Do to Prevent Photosensitivity

Not everyone who takes a photoreactive drug will experience a reaction. Nonetheless, it is important to take some precautions if your doctor has prescribed a medicine with the side effect of photosensitivity. To prevent, or reduce the likelihood, of a reaction, take the following measures:

◊ Use a sunscreen with an SPF of 15 or higher. Make sure your sunscreen is free of PABA, which can trigger a photosensitive reaction.

◊ Wear protective clothing such as a wide-brimmed hat.

◊ Avoid prolonged periods of sun exposure, including the use of tanning booths.

◊ If you're fair-skinned, it's best to avoid sunlight altogether while taking the drug in question.

◊ Ask your physician if an alternative medication— one that does not cause a photosensitive reaction—can be prescribed.

◊ Consider supplementing with natural *photoprotective agents*. A number of nutritional substances have been found in research to protect the skin against the harmful effects of ultraviolet rays. These substances include dietary fish oil, green tea, and beta-carotene. Other photoprotective agents are vitamins C and E. When taken together, vitamin C (2 grams daily) and vitamin E (1,000 IU daily) reduced the severity of sunburn significantly, according to one study. Before supplementing, however, check with your doctor.

◊ Ask your doctor or pharmacist if a drug you're taking will trigger photosensitivity. Further, always read the directions that come with any medicine to see if it can cause problems.

4

Youth-Enhancing Moisturizers

I T starts out with tiny, white scales. Then comes flaking, cracking, and possibly some chapping. You've got dry skin, and it makes you look like you've seen better days.

Medically known as *xerosis,* dry skin is distinguished by a lack of moisture in the outer portion of the epidermis, the stratum corneum. With age, skin dries out because of the shrinkage in oil and sweat glands as well as a slowdown in the turnover of epidermal cells. These cells remain on the surface, partially attached to skin, and appear as scales. Dry skin is less flexible, rough in texture, and, unfortunately, more vulnerable to wrinkles.

Under normal conditions, your face and the rest of your skin are moisturized and lubricated naturally, day in and day out. Delivered to skin cells by tiny blood vessels, water moves up from the dermis to the stratum corneum and hydrates the cells. This type of water, which originates from within the body, is termed *transepidermal water* and is the most effective source of water for hydrating skin. Eventually, transepidermal water evaporates into the air. Sweat glands also help keep the skin naturally moist.

The rate of transepidermal water loss depends largely on a collection of water-attracting and water-retaining nutrients in the stratum corneum known as the *natural moisturizing factor* (NMF). The NMF includes amino acids, pyrolidone carboxylic acid (PCA), lactates, urea, and minerals. They work together to reduce evaporation and keep the skin naturally moisturized. Aged skin contains less NMF than younger skin. Water-attracting PCA, in particular, declines by half in older skin.

Besides aging, other factors can accelerate water loss from the stratum corneum. These include cool weather with low humidity; air-conditioning; frequent bathing; overuse of soap; heredity; and diseases such as an underactive thyroid. When water loss is rapid, skin cells become irregularly shaped, and cell walls weaken. Fine lines and cracks readily develop on dry skin.

Although dry skin is associated mostly with the stratum corneum, the dermis is involved to a lesser extent. There are water-holding proteins called *glycosaminoglycans* (GAGs) in the dermis that help moisturize your skin. But GAGs decline with age, leaving less natural moisture underneath.

Skin is lubricated by the secretion of sebum from your oil glands. The oil acts as a natural barrier to prevent too much water from escaping. But as you get older, your sweat and oil glands wither, robbing your skin of this natural source of lubrication and protection.

In the stratum corneum, there is also a special group of lipids, arranged in a layered matrix that binds corneocytes together. They regulate the skin's water balance and help prevent water from leaving the skin. These lipids, which decline with age, include ceramides, cholesterol, and essential fatty acids.

Other factors are at work, too. If you're undergoing menopause—the natural stage in life that marks the end of your reproductive years—your supply of collagen begins to diminish. Collagen not only gives your skin its resiliency, it also takes up water to moisturize the skin. With age, collagen loses this moisturizing ability, leaving skin rough and brittle. In addition, your body is producing less estrogen—a hormonal decline that dries out your skin.

So you see, with age and other factors, you become especially vulnerable to dry skin—and the wrinkles that accompany it.

MOISTURIZERS 911

Moisturizers are cosmetics that improve the condition of the skin by increasing the water content in the stratum corneum. They relieve dry skin in three broad ways—by working as occlusives, humectants, and emollients. Most products are formulated with a combination of all three types of moisturizers, plus other skin-friendly ingredients.

Occlusives

Occlusives are agents that, when applied topically, act as a barrier against moisture to entrap the skin's moisture loss from the skin. They do this primarily by remaining on the skin's surface, without being absorbed. This action prevents transepidermal water loss, boosts the water content in the stratum corneum, and smoothes the rough texture of dry skin. As a result, skin becomes softer and more flexible. Overall skin appearance is improved, too. A downside of occlusives is that they sometimes feel heavy and greasy on the skin.

Occlusive agents include petroleum jelly (petrolatum), lanolin, jojoba oil, cocoa butter, paraffin, cholesterol, olive oil, and mineral oil. Of these, one of the best is petroleum jelly because it does a superior job of reducing transepidermal water loss.

Humectants

Humectants are ingredients that can attract water from the environment and natural moisture from underlying skin tissue. They have the power to retain up to a thousand times their weight in water—a property that plumps up the skin, making it appear smoother.

Common humectants found in moisturizers include glycerin, sorbitol, sodium lactate, hyaluronic acid, and PCA. Alpha hydroxy acids are another humectant, better known for their ability to slough off dead skin cells. Alpha hydroxy acids are discussed in chapter 6.

A very effective humectant is urea, also a component of the skin's natural moisturizing factor (NMF). It works by breaking apart hydrogen bonds in the molecular structure of the skin's surface. This allows corneocytes to become "unglued" so that their water-binding sites are exposed. Water molecules can thus flow into those sites to allow the skin's surface to retain more water.

Humectants feel lighter and less greasy on the skin than occlusives.

Emollients

Emollients pack the spaces between dry skin flakes with oil, smoothing the rough surface of the stratum corneum. They have little or no influence on transepidermal water loss. Examples of emollients include vitamin E, fatty acids, and squalane. If applied heavily, many emollients function as occlusives.

Other Moisturizing Ingredients

In addition to the occlusives, humectants, or emollients, here's a look at some of the more common cosmetic additives you find in moisturizers:

Water. Water is a major ingredient of most moisturizers, although it tends to evaporate shortly after application. Most moisturizers are formulated as either oil-in-water or water-in-oil emulsions. Oil-in-water moisturizers tend to be oilier and feel greasier, but they remain on the skin longer. Water-in-oil moisturizers are lighter and less greasy, but rub off more easily.

Cosmetic natural moisturizing factor (NMF). Companies have sought to approximate the skin's NMF by formulating their products with cosmetic versions of nutrients found in the skin: amino acids, lactic acid, urea, and various minerals. Lactic acid, in particular, has been found to reduce the roughness of dry, chapped skin on the face. PCA is a NMF component found in numerous moisturizers, and one that has been shown to do an excellent job of restoring the skin's water content. A problem with the use of individual components of the NMF, however, is that they are very water soluble. When you cleanse your skin, they wash off easily, and their benefits do not last very long.

Lipids. Numerous commercially available moisturizers are formulated with lipids (fats and oils) as their active ingredients. Studies show that applying skin-identical lipids significantly improves the "barrier function" of skin. This simply means that the lipids prevent an excessive amount of water from leaving the skin.

A common lipid found in moisturizers is a cosmetic form of ceramides, which in their natural state are constituents of the stratum corneum. These cosmetic versions mimic the skin's own lipids and have proven effective in preventing water loss from the skin. They do not, however, stimulate the skin to create a new supply of natural ceramides.

Natural oils such as almond, olive, safflower, and sunflower are also found in moisturizers. They can dissolve in sebum and are thus readily absorbed by skin cells.

Liposomes. Marketed by cosmetic companies since the mid-1980s, liposomes are tiny sacs that carry hydrating ingredients to skin cells. Supposedly, they are small enough to seep into the stratum corneum, but skin researchers assert that they do not penetrate that layer and therefore are incapable of truly moisturizing the skin. Liposomes, however, coat the surface of the skin, allowing humectants to stay on the skin longer.

Vitamins. Many moisturizers are enriched with small doses of various vitamins, namely vitamin A, vitamin C, and vitamin E. All are antioxidants that when applied topically may help prevent or reduce free-radical damage to the skin. They are often combined in commercial moisturizers. Vitamin E, in particular, is an emollient with a proven ability to moisturize the skin. For more information on skin vitamins, see chapter 7.

Botanicals. Among the botanicals (herbs) found in some moisturizers are chamomile, believed to have a soothing effect on skin; aloe vera, which has a repairing effect on damaged skin; and seaweeds, which help the skin retain moisture. Other moisture-providing botanicals include mulberry, licorice, and thyme. For more information on botanicals, see chapter 8; for information on seaweed and other marine products, refer to chapter 9.

Collagen. A number of moisturizers are formulated with collagen, and claims have been made that it replaces the old, degenerated collagen in the skin. This claim is not true, however. The collagen molecule is so large that it cannot penetrate the stratum corneum. "This would be like trying to put a basketball through a hole the size of a Ping-Pong ball," wrote Richard F. Wehr and Lincoln Krochmal, M.D., in the medical journal *Cutis*.

However, there is a benefit to using a moisturizer formulated with collagen or other cosmetic proteins such as elastin, keratin, or hydrolysates (water-bound proteins). Like mortar, they fill in the irregularities on the surface of dry skin. Plus, they coat the skin with a film that keeps moisture in. This film may shrink a bit as they dry on the face, smoothing out wrinkles temporarily.

Elastin. The rubberlike protein elastin is often combined with collagen in commercial moisturizers. Skin researchers, however, feel that because the stratum corneum cannot properly absorb it, elastin does not have any effect on the skin. Like collagen, however, elastin coats the skin and helps lock in moisture. It fills in surface irregularities as well.

Glycosaminoglycans (GAGs). These water-holding proteins are present as hydrolysates in moisturizers. But as yet, there are no studies to verify a moisturizing benefit when added to a skin-care product. Like other cosmetic proteins, however, they help temporarily fill in cracks and flaws in the skin's surface.

Emulsifiers. The job of emulsifiers is to hold the water and oil in a lotion in suspension. Emulsifiers also keep water in the skin. Common emulsifiers are lecithin, stearic acid, and stearyl alcohol.

Solvents. The role of solvents in moisturizers is to help dissolve other ingredients in the formulation. A commonly used solvent is propylene glycol, which also serves as a humectant.

Another solvent is alcohol. When you apply your moisturizer, alcohol provides a cooling effect caused by its rapid evaporation. In higher concentrations, however, alcohol can cause skin problems, particularly if your skin is on the dry side.

Sunscreens. Many facial moisturizers contain sunscreen agents, which protect the skin against the harmful effects of ultraviolet light and thus minimize the chance of developing wrinkles. For more information on sunscreens, see chapter 3.

Noncomedogenic moisturizers. These are products containing ingredients that won't plug up your pores. The label of a moisturizer will state whether it is noncomedogenic.

Fragrances and preservatives. Fragrances mask the odor of the formulation and impart a pleasing smell to the moisturizer. However, some fragrances provoke untoward reactions, and many women are sensitive or even allergic to them. According to an article published in the journal *Dermatologic Nursing,* 65 percent of moisturizers on the market contain fragrances.

Preservatives are essential to moisturizers, particularly those formulated with water, because they prevent bacterial contamination. But like fragrances, some preservatives are irritants. A common preservative in facial moisturizers is a group of substances called *parabens,* usually methyl paraben and propyl paraben. Paraben mixtures have been known to cause allergic reactions in sensitive skin.

If you have sensitive skin, test a moisturizer before buying it. Apply a little bit to your neck, leave it on for a while, and see how it reacts with your skin.

MOISTURIZERS AND WRINKLES

Moisturizers are not antiwrinkle products per se. Nor can manufacturers, by law, make wrinkle-removing claims for their moisturizers. They can't state in any way that moisturizers will alter the structure or function of the skin.

Manufacturers can, however, say that their products "diminish," "ease," or "minimize" fine lines and wrinkles. Indeed, the routine use of facial moisturizers does have a positive effect on wrinkled skin—in four impressive ways.

First, they treat dry skin. Moisturizers work at the level of the stratum corneum and normally do not penetrate below that layer of skin. But that is where moisturizers are most needed. Deeper layers of skin don't dry out like the stratum corneum does. Keeping the stratum corneum moisturized is vital for protecting its integrity and normal function.

Second, by hydrating the skin, facial moisturizers plump

it up. This minimizes and improves the appearance of wrinkles.

Third, moisturizers act as temporary "fillers." The solid material found in moisturizers fills in the tiny crevices of wrinkles, making the skin look smoother. Of course, this is only a temporary benefit, lasting six to eight hours, but it improves the overall appearance of wrinkled skin nonetheless.

Fourth, some moisturizers contain cosmetically inactive ingredients that reflect light away your face, making wrinkles less noticeable to people looking at you.

WHICH MOISTURIZER IS BEST?

With thousands of moisturizers on the market, this is a question which is nearly impossible to answer! However, there is research that can steer you in the right direction.

In my opinion, the most helpful research conducted on moisturizers was published in *Consumers Reports* in January 2000. The *Consumers Report* testers examined 28 lotions and creams, 12 of which were formulated for the face. They noted that the facial moisturizers did not vary much in their ingredients, but that there was a wide swing in price—from $1.40 to $33 per ounce.

The testers selected 30 subjects and conducted the research in a lab under tightly controlled conditions. They applied moisturizers to the subjects' calves, where the skin is very similar to facial skin. Using a special instrument called a Corneometer, the testers measured skin moisture before the product was applied, one hour after application, two hours after, and four hours after. The products were also evaluated by how they felt on the skin—heavy or light, thick or thin, well absorbed or not well absorbed, and so forth.

Now for the results: Two facial moisturizers won hands down. They were L'Oréal Plentitude Active Daily Moisture at $1.59 an ounce and Pond's Nourishing Moisturizer at $1.40 an ounce—two of the least expensive moisturizers, which goes to show that pricey is not always best when it comes to cosmetics. According to the research report, both products produced "large, long-lasting increases in moisture level." In addition, both products have an SPF of 15.

In choosing a moisturizer, dermatologist Albert M. Kligman, M.D., Ph.D., offers this helpful advice in the *Journal of Women's Health & Gender-Based Medicine:* "I recommend products that have only a few basic ingredients, such as petrolatum, mineral oil, and other time-tested emollients, and that have been around a long time. One example is Nivea cream (Beiersdorf, Inc., Norwalk, Connecticut), which is an excellent moisturizer that contains only four ingredients. The fewer the ingredients, the less is the likelihood of skin reactions and irritation."

GETTING THE MOST FROM YOUR MOISTURIZER

Regardless of which moisturizer you select, there are ways to maximize its moisturizing properties, plus minimize the potential for dry skin. For example:

◊ Use warm—not hot—water when you bathe or shower. Hot water has a drying effect on skin.

◊ Use a nonsoap cleanser on your face. Harsh soaps can dry out skin, plus aggravate already dry skin.

◊ Pat your face after washing. Leave your skin slightly moist.

◊ Apply moisturizer immediately after washing your face and patting it. This helps lock in additional moisture and keeps water from evaporating.

◊ Because a moisturizer will rub off during the day, apply it twice daily—in the morning and evening.

◊ Drink eight to 10 full glasses of water daily to keep the skin and other body tissues well hydrated.

◊ Cut down on alcohol and caffeine. Both substances act as diuretics; that is, they promote water loss from the body, including skin cells.

◊ Quit smoking. It dries the skin, plus makes it leathery and wrinkled.

◊ Work with a skin-care professional to help you select the best moisturizer for your skin type.

PART THREE

Skin Rejuvenators

5

The Remarkable Retinoids

UNLESS you've been stranded on a desert island, you've heard about the antiwrinkle products Retin-A and Renova. These are the best known of the topical *retinoids,* a group of compounds derived from vitamin A, a nutrient that has been used as a therapeutic agent in dermatology for more than fifty years. It is essential for normal skin growth and maintenance.

Some retinoids are natural derivatives of vitamin A. Others, like Retin-A and Renova, are chemical copies, or synthetic versions, of the natural forms. To date, the pharmaceutical industry has synthesized approximately 2,500 new retinoids. Both the natural and synthetic agents have the power to successfully treat numerous skin problems, including facial wrinkles and photoaging.

RETIN-A AND RENOVA

Retin-A and Renova are known generically as *tretinoin,* which was first tested in 1959 as a treatment for skin diseases. Later, Retin-A was developed as an acne drug by the prominent dermatologist Alfred M. Kligman, M.D., Ph.D., at the University of Pennsylvania School of Medicine. It was launched as a prescription medicine for acne in 1971 and is manufactured by Ortho Pharmaceuticals. A newer form of the drug, Retin-A Micro, was introduced in 1996. It houses tretinoin in microscopic particles called *microsponges* that allow for a slow, time-release delivery to reduce skin irritation.

After Retin-A's introduction in the seventies, older patients using it for acne began to notice that the drug not only cured pimples, but also smoothed out the fine lines on their faces, made freckles fade, and gave their skin a rosy glow. Consequently, Dr. Kligman began his pioneering and now famous work on the antiwrinkle benefits of Retin-A. Many clinical trials followed, the majority of which reaching the same conclusion: Retin-A truly does improve the appearance of aging skin.

By 1988, Retin-A had gained fame as an antiwrinkle cream, although it was not (and still isn't) approved for that use by the FDA. Even so, many dermatologists have continued to prescribe it for patients who want to erase facial wrinkles and rejuvenate their skin. This practice—known as an "off-label indication"—is perfectly legal. Retin-A, however, can't be promoted as an antiwrinkle medication.

Ortho Pharmaceuticals reformulated and tested Retin-A under the brand name Renova as a bona fide antiwrinkle product. In 1995, it was approved by the FDA for enhancing the appearance of photodamaged skin, minimizing wrinkles, reducing roughness, and improving the overall texture of skin. Renova is a less irritating form of tretinoin because it comes in a rich, cosmeticlike emollient base made from light mineral oil, purified water, and other ingredients.

Whereas Retin-A and Retin-A Micro are indicated for

treating acne, Renova is designed specifically for wrinkled, aging skin. You need a prescription from your physician or dermatologist to use these medications.

HOW DO RETIN-A AND RENOVA WORK?

Neither is a cosmetic. They are drugs because their active ingredient—tretinoin—alters the structure and function of the skin by affecting skin-cell growth in the epidermal and dermal layers. The net result is to reverse the effects of both intrinsic and extrinsic aging in the skin. Specifically, tretinoin:

Boosts Collagen Production

Collagen is the bodily protein that keeps your skin firm and taut. But with age and increased activity of free radicals, normal collagen production declines and skin loses its youthful strength and firmness. Tretinoin, however, stimulates the formation of new collagen, resulting in greater firmness. It also restores elasticity so that your skin retains its suppleness and ability to bounce back when stretched.

Tretinoin also appears to prevent the destruction of collagen and elastin. Some studies have found that tretinoin blocks the action of *metalloproteinases,* enzymes triggered by ultraviolet radiation that destroy collagen and elastin.

Reduces the Number and Depth of Wrinkles

The power of tretinoin to reduce skin wrinkling associated with photodamage has been well studied. Case in point: In one six-month study, patients applied a 0.025 percent concentration of tretinoin. Afterward, they began using a 0.05 percent concentration. Researchers checked the patients every month and then again every four months. Over the course of the experiment, the number of wrinkles and the depth of wrinkles were reduced. Brown spots on the skin faded as well.

Preserves the Natural Density of Skin

Tretinoin thickens the top layer (the epidermis) of your skin, making it look more compact. This benefit means that tretinoin is an excellent medication for older skin that has thinned out as a natural outcome of the aging process.

Generates New Blood Vessels

With age, we tend to lose blood vessels in our skin, and the net effect is a pale complexion. Using tretinoin promotes *angiogenesis,* the formation of new blood vessels in the skin for improved blood flow. This imparts the characteristic rosy glow seen in the complexions of people who use Retin-A or Renova. With increased blood flow, the skin is better supplied with the nutrients, fluids, and oxygen it requires for repair and maintenance. Stepping up circulation also clears away toxic substances that would otherwise compromise the integrity of the skin.

Reduces Pore Size

Remember how your skin looked at age nine or ten? In all likelihood, your pores were barely visible, giving your complexion a velvetlike appearance. Later in life, though, pores enlarge as impacted corneocytes and bundles of fine hairs become entrapped within them. Bacteria and yeasts breed inside the pores, further dilating them.

For such problems, tretinoin is a white knight of sorts. It removes these impurities from your pores and thus shrinks pore size, turning the clock back to younger-looking skin.

Increases Cell Turnover

Exfoliation—the removal of dead cells from the skin's surface—has become an important skin-care issue. When skin is exfoliated, it takes on a softer, smoother, more uniform appearance. Tretinoin exfoliates by sloughing off skin-dulling dead cells.

Bleaches Freckles and Blotches

As a slougher, tretinoin also helps alleviate unsightly skin discoloration. Among the cells sloughed off the skin by tretinoin are melanin-filled keratinocytes, which cause freckling and age spots. When these pigmented cells are shed, skin color becomes more uniform, and there is less blotchiness.

WHICH STRENGTH WORKS BEST?

Renova contains a 0.05 percent concentration of tretinoin. Retin-A cream comes in three strengths: 0.1 percent, 0.05 percent, and 0.025 percent. It is also available as a gel, either as a 0.025 percent or 0.01 percent strength. There is also a liquid version of Retin-A, which contains 0.05 percent tretinoin. Retin-A Micro is formulated as a 0.1 percent concentration of tretinoin.

Studies indicate that tretinoin at any strength between 0.025 and 0.1 percent improves the severity of photoaging and reduces wrinkles. Although you may get faster results with the highest concentration (0.1 percent), you could endure more side effects, such as skin irritation. Your dermatologist may start you out on a low-dose 0.025 percent tretinoin cream and gradually increase the dose to a 0.05 percent cream, depending on how well your skin tolerates the medication.

Using Renova and Retin-A

Your dermatologist will give you specific instructions on how to apply these medications, depending on which one is prescribed for your particular situation. Some dermatologists prefer Retin-A for aging skin because it is available in stronger concentrations.

Whatever the case, tretinoin should be applied at night prior to bedtime—for two reasons. First, sunlight can degrade tretinoin. Second, nightly application allows the medication to remain undisturbed on the skin.

Before applying the medication, remove all makeup and thoroughly cleanse your skin with a gentle soap or alcohol-free cleanser. Wait 20 to 30 minutes before applying the medication to make sure your skin is completely dry. (Wet, damp, or moist skin absorbs the cream too rapidly and may lead to irritation.) Squeeze a pea-sized dab of the cream on each temple and spread it over your entire face. According to Dr. Kligman, it is perfectly safe to apply the cream around your eyelids where fine wrinkles are so evident, even though package directions caution against it.

Writing in the medical journal *Cutis,* he noted: "I show patients how to make the applications right up to the lid margins and vermilion borders of the lips. Except for short-lived stinging, no harm results from tretinoin getting into the eyes and mouth."

The following morning, cleanse your face to remove any residual cream. Because tretinoin is an exfoliating agent, your skin may become dry and slightly scaly. To combat these potential side effects, apply a non-pore-clogging moisturizer to your skin in the morning. Dr. Kligman recommends Nivea Ultra Moisturizing Crème and Eucerin creams (not the lotions), as well as petroleum jelly or the creamy version of Vasoline. Moisturizers containing lanolin are also effective. If needed, the moisturizer should be reapplied in the afternoon.

While using tretinoin, avoid the following: facial scrubs; toners or astringents containing alcohol; and waxing, depilatories or bleach on facial hair. These will irritate your skin.

Continue to apply the cream daily for eight months to a year. Afterward, you can cut back to a Monday, Wednesday, Friday maintenance regimen. To maintain the benefits, continue to use tretinoin indefinitely, for life.

WHAT ARE THE SIDE EFFECTS?

With initial use, you may experience some mild redness, swelling, or scaliness. These can be alleviated with the use of a hydrocortisone cream, applied along with tretinoin, for a few days. Within a few weeks, however, these side effects will subside as your skin becomes acclimated to the medication.

In the early stages of use, tretinoin makes your skin more sensitive to sunlight, and you may sunburn more easily. That being so, avoid noonday sun, apply sunscreen with a SPF of 15 or more, shun tanning booths, and wear sun-protective clothing. After a few months of using tretinoin, this enhanced sensitivity to sunlight will virtually disappear.

Worth noting, too, is that extremes of weather, such as wind or cold, may be more irritating to your skin when you are using this medication.

Tretinoin has not been linked negatively in any way to the risk of cancer. The drug has been used by millions of patients worldwide for more than 30 years. In fact, emerging new research indicates that tretinoin may help prevent skin cancer.

Tretinoin should always be used under medical supervision.

ACCORDING TO THE
PHYSICIANS' DESK REFERENCE,
DO NOT USE TRETINOIN IF:

◊ You have any type of skin disease.

◊ Your skin is red, inflamed, infected, or otherwise irritated.

◊ You are sensitive to or have ever had an allergic reaction to tretinoin.

◊ You are pregnant or plan to become pregnant.

◊ You are lactating. (It is not known whether the drug appears in breast milk.)

◊ You are taking drugs that make your skin more sensitive to sunlight.

HOW LONG WILL IT TAKE TO SEE RESULTS?

You should begin to see smoother, softer skin in about a month. Over the next four to five months, lines, wrinkles, and brown spots will begin to fade. Other benefits such as firmer, thicker skin will materialize in about five months. Plus, with every year that you continue to apply tretinoin, more new collagen is deposited in your skin, and your complexion will continue to improve.

OVER-THE-COUNTER RETINOIDS

Natural retinoids that are available in over-the-counter formulations include retinol and retinyl palmitate (also known as retinol palmitate).

Retinol is the pure form of vitamin A. In the past, topical retinol was too "unstable" to exert any antiwrinkle benefits. Once it touched the skin, retinol would break down and become inactive.

Recently, though, scientists have developed more stable preparations, and clinical trials with retinol as a skin rejuvenator have been impressive. Some studies have found that retinol, in appropriate concentrations, is as effective as tretinoin and much less irritating. It has been found to thicken the epidermal layer, plus regenerate collagen in aging skin.

Case in point: In a recent study conducted at the University of Michigan, researchers looked into the effects of topical retinol (a 1 percent solution) applied to the skin of volunteers aged 80 or older. The researchers were interested in learning whether retinol was effective on naturally aged skin, as opposed to photodamaged skin, so they selected sites that had been protected from the sun. What they discovered was remarkable: Retinol blocked the action of collagen-degrading enzymes (metalloproteinases) and stimulated the production of new collagen—and did so in just seven days!

Like tretinoin, retinol is an exfoliant. It accelerates the process by which dead skin cells are sloughed off, thus smoothing and retexturizing the skin.

In addition, retinol is an *antioxidant,* a nutrient that squelches free radicals and prevents them from doing harm. When applied topically, retinol is believed to help protect skin cells against free-radical damage. (For more information on other topical antioxidants, see chapter 7.)

Numerous cosmetic products are formulated with retinol. However, it is difficult to determine exact concentration, and many products contain minute quantities of retinol. For treating wrinkles and photoaging, though, tretinoin is still preferred by dermatologists and physicians. It works much better because it is stronger than most retinol products.

Another retinoid found in cosmetics is retinyl palmitate, which is about half as potent as pure retinol. Most dermatologists caution that retinyl palmitate is topically ineffective. However, it appears to work well against very dry skin. So does another retinol—retinyl linoleate.

As yet, there are no studies proving the effectiveness of these forms of retinols against wrinkles or other symptoms of skin aging. The lesson here: Carefully read the labels of any over-the-counter retinoid product so that you know which type of retinol you're buying.

6

Skin-Smoothing Hydroxy Acids

I once asked a prominent dermatologist—whose skin was flawless—what she recommended for a wrinkle-free complexion. Her answer: sunscreen and alpha hydroxy acids.

Why such a resounding endorsement for alpha hydroxy acids (AHAs)? Because AHAs and other hydroxy acids have skin-rejuvenating benefits galore. They exfoliate dead skin cells, moisturize the skin, thicken the dermis, repair damage caused by sunlight, and quite possibly stimulate collagen-making processes in the skin.

Alpha hydroxy acids are mild organic acids found in nature. (Acids, in general, are compounds that release hydrogen in a watery solution.) There are several varieties of AHAs in cosmetics. The most frequently used is glycolic acid, found in honey or sugarcane. Others are lactic acid, derived from sour milk or mangoes; malic acid, from apples or pears; citric acid from lemons or oranges; and tartaric acid, from fermented grapes. However, most AHAs used in cosmetics are man-made.

Long before AHAs were chemically isolated and their

skin-smoothing benefits recognized, they were used as cosmetics. When Cleopatra took milk baths, she was unknowingly treating her skin with lactic acid. Women of the French court washed their faces in old wine, which contains tartaric acid. Your grandmother may have applied a mask of honey or mashed fruit to her face, without ever realizing that the mask was filled with skin-rejuvenating ingredients we know today as AHAs.

The use of AHAs in dermatology was discovered in 1974 when two researchers found that these acids could be used to treat an inherited skin disease called *ichthyosis*. It is characterized by dry skin, with a fish-scale appearance. The researchers, who coined the term *alpha hydroxy acids,* observed that AHAs effectively sloughed off dead skin cells to alleviate the scaliness. Later, in 1984, the same researchers found that wrinkles were gradually reduced in patients using lactic acid to treat keratoses, tiny benign wartlike growths on the skin.

Eventually, dermatologists and plastic surgeons developed the "chemical peel," a strong concentration of alpha hydroxy acids that, when applied to the face, helps remove the unattractive signs of aging such as wrinkles, roughness, and blotches.

Around 1992, cosmetic manufacturers began mass-marketing skin-care products containing milder concentrations of the acids found in chemical peels. These products catapulted into popularity. At last count, there were approximately 45 companies, manufacturing more than 200 different alpha hydroxy products, from over-the-counter lotions or creams to chemical peels used by dermatologists and plastic surgeons. Worldwide sales have now exceeded $1 billion. Cleansers, creams, lotions, gels, and astringents are among the products formulated with AHAs. The number of alpha hydroxy products on the market continues to mushroom.

The term *alpha hydroxy* refers to the chemical structure

of the acid. In scientific lingo, AHAs have one hydroxyl group attached to the first carbon following the acid group, designated as *alpha* after the first letter of the Greek alphabet.

A cosmetic acid similar to AHAs is one known as *beta hydroxy* (BHA). Structurally, BHAs are molecules in which the hydroxy group is on the second carbon next to the acid group, hence the designation *beta* for the second letter of the Greek alphabet. The most widely used BHA in certain antiwrinkle cosmetics is salicylic acid, a derivative of aspirin. When applied topically, both AHAs and BHAs work in the same fashion, and the end result is to erase the undesirable marks of skin aging and revitalize aging skin. (See table 6.1 for a list of AHAs and BHAs found in cosmetics.)

THE RIGHT FORMULATION FOR YOUR FACE

When deciding on which hydroxy acid product to use, there are three factors to consider: its concentration of AHAs or BHAs; its pH; and the vehicle of the formulation. All three factors influence the product's effectiveness.

Concentration

The concentration of hydroxy acids in a product's solution is expressed as a percentage. For example, most hydroxy products sold over-the-counter usually contain acid concentrations of 10 percent or less. Generally, higher-concentration hydroxy preparations deliver more desirable results. If the concentration is too little, there won't be much effect on skin at all. The concentration may or may not be stated on the product label.

Table 6.1: Hydroxy Acids in Cosmetics

ALPHA HYDROXY ACIDS	BETA HYDROXY ACIDS
Glycolic acid	Salicylic acid
Lactic acid	Beta hydroxybutanoic
Malic acid	acid
Mandelic acid	Tropic acid
Citric acid	Trethocanic acid
Tartaric acid	
Glycolic acid + ammonia glycolate	
Alpha-hydroxyethanoic acid + ammonium alpha-hydroxyethanoate	
Alpha-hydroxyoctanoic acid	
Alpha-hydroxycaprylic acid	
Hydroxycaprylic acid	
Mixed fruit acid	
Triple fruit acid	
Tri-alpha hydroxy fruit acids	
Sugarcane extract	
Alpha hydroxy and botanical complex	
l-alpha hydroxy acid	
Glycomer in cross-linked fatty acids alpha nutrium	

Source: The Food and Drug Administration. 1999. Alpha hydroxy acids for skin care: smooth sailing or rough seas. *The FDA Consumer*. March–April. Online: www.fda.gov.

pH

The strength of an acid solution is expressed as its pH. In essence, pH measures acidity on a point scale. A solution with a pH of 1 is a strong acid; and one with a pH of 7 is neutral. A solution having a pH of 14 is considered to be a strong "base" (bases are the opposite of acids). Put another way, the higher the pH, the weaker the acid.

What many women don't realize is that with hydroxy products, pH is more important than concentration. Here's why: The lower (or more acidic) the pH, the better its absorption and the greater its exfoliating action. Lower pH formulations, however, tend to be more irritating to the skin.

Over-the-counter preparations contain hydroxy acids with a pH of 2 to 8, although most are either 3 to 4. In tests with these acids, a pH of 3 was found to best stimulate the turnover and renewal of skin cells. Also, AHAs with a pH of 6 or greater behave more like moisturizers than like exfoliants.

Dermatologists generally recommend using an over-the-counter hydroxy product with a concentration of 10 percent and a pH of 3.5 or greater. Among the few that fall into this category is Aqua Glycolic, manufactured by Merz Pharmaceuticals. Billed as having the highest concentration of glycolic acid without a prescription, Aqua Glycolic is available at most major pharmacies and mass-market retailers like Wal-Mart. At some pharmacies, it is a "behind-the-counter" product. You have to ask the pharmacist for it, even though it doesn't require a prescription. Aqua Glycolic costs about $12 for a two-ounce bottle.

As with concentration, the pH may or may not be listed on the label. There's an easy way to self-test the product's strength, though. When applied, does it tingle? If not, it probably isn't strong enough.

Solutions intended for use in salons and in dermatologic or plastic surgery clinics are stronger than those available over-the-counter. In salons, for example, where you can have mild glycolic-acid facials, solutions vary in concentration—from 4 to 50 percent. As with over-the-counter products, the pH is generally 2 to 8. Products used by physicians for chemical peels are even stronger, with a pH of 2 or less and concentrations ranging from 4 to 67 percent.

While most hydroxy products are classified by the FDA as cosmetics, there is one exception: Lac-Hydrin, a prescription AHA drug manufactured by Westwood-Squibb Pharmaceutical. Lac-Hydrin contains 12 percent lactic acid and ammonium lactate and has a pH ranging from 4.5 to 5.5. Dermatologists prescribe it for dry skin and to treat sun-damaged skin.

Lac-Hydrin works near miracles against wrinkles and skin roughness. In one study, 21 volunteers applied the lotion twice daily to their skin for eight weeks. Within four weeks, skin improvements were readily noticeable. And by the end of the experimental period, there was mild to moderate improvement in wrinkles in 15 patients. What's more, their skin was visibly softer and smoother. For information about Lac-Hydrin, talk to your physician or dermatologist.

Vehicle

The "vehicle" refers to the carrier substance, such as a cream or lotion, into which the hydroxy acid is mixed. Because hydroxy acids are water soluble, they are normally mixed in purified water or in creams or lotions of oil-in-water emulsions.

The vehicle plays an important role in the effectiveness of the product, particularly as it pertains to different skin types. Let's say your skin is on the dry side. Then it's best to choose an emollient cream, which can help restore your skin's natural balance of oil and water. If your skin is normal to oily, lotions are your best bet. For oily, acne-prone skin, try an alcohol-based formulation, which is less likely to clog pores.

HOW DO AHAS AND BHAS WORK?

By FDA definition, AHAs and BHAs are cosmetics, even though they are similar to drugs in some respects. Cosmetics that act like drugs are termed *cosmeceuticals* in the skin-care industry. So it's safe to say that hydroxy acids are cosmeceuticals.

Cosmetically, AHAs and BHAs have important functional advantages, even though skin researchers do not yet know exactly how they work. What's more, their benefits are backed by mounds of scientific data. Hydroxy acids:

Increase Exfoliation

As your skin ages, the turnover of epidermal (upper-layer) cells decelerates. These dead cells tend to clump together on the skin's surface rather than getting sloughed off, and your facial skin begins to appear dull and feel rough. To make your skin look smoother again, you should exfoliate your complexion—that is, remove those dead skin cells.

There are various ways to exfoliate. These include mechanical methods such as scrubbing with a loofah sponge or special exfoliation sponges; or chemical means such as using AHAs or BHAs or having a chemical peel. As chemical exfoliants, AHAs and BHAs penetrate the living skin tissue, then unglue and detach dead skin cells (corneocytes) on the outer layer of the epidermis. This accelerates cell division in the deeper layer of the epidermis (the stratum basale). The normal process of skin-cell regeneration thus speeds up, resulting in fresher, more youthful-looking skin.

Over-the-counter AHA and BHA cosmetics do an admirable job of exfoliation. For more intense exfoliation, you may want to consider a chemical peel, particularly if you have very deep wrinkles. Information on chemical peels is found in chapter 10.

Stimulate Collagen Production

Until quite recently, it was believed that hydroxy acids were incapable of rebuilding collagen, the protein that keeps your skin firm. But emerging research is beginning to show otherwise. AHAs, in particular, do indeed stimulate the production of collagen. In experiments in which scientists placed fibroblasts from skin tissue in lab dishes and treated them with glycolic acid, a common AHA, the fibroblasts began producing more collagen.

Concentration makes a difference in collagen synthesis, too. Studies have found that a 20 percent concentration of AHA results in significant collagen production. But to a lesser extent, so do concentrations of 5, 10, and 15 percent.

Scientists speculate that AHAs rebuild collagen in the skin through a mechanism somehow related to ascorbic acid (vitamin C). One of ascorbic acid's chief duties in the body is to stimulate the growth of collagen. Ascorbic acid is chemically derived from an AHA, so perhaps the connection lies in the functional similarities between the two.

Improve Sagging Skin

As your skin matures, the dermis begins to thin out. This can lead to sagging skin, as well as to wrinkles, papery skin, and overall loss of skin integrity. Using hydroxy acids, however, picks up the slack on sagging skin and reverses other undesirable changes in your skin. Hydroxy acids do so by thickening your skin.

Within the first three months of use, hydroxy acids can

increase the thickness of the dermis, according to a number of studies. This newly acquired thickness appears to be caused by three favorable changes in skin proteins. First, there is an increase in GAGs (glycosaminoglycans), water-binding proteins in skin that keep it smooth and supple. Normally, GAGs decline with age. Second, new collagen is formed in the dermis. And third, the quality of the skin's elastin fibers is improved.

Reduce Photoaging

Skin that has been damaged by chronic sun exposure appears dry and yellowish, with wrinkles and a coarse texture. As noted earlier, dermatologists and skin specialists refer to this condition as *photoaging*.

Quite a few studies indicate that hydroxy acids can repair photoaged skin. Researchers found that women who used either 8 percent glycolic acid, 8 percent lactic acid, or a placebo on their faces for 22 weeks achieved at least one grade of improvement in the overall severity of photoaging. One experiment found that even a very mild AHA (5 percent glycolic acid) noticeably reduced skin roughness, compared with a placebo cream.

Chronic sun exposure also produces brownish discolorations on the skin. When combined with lightening agents such as hydroquinone, AHAs are very effective at bleaching brown spots and other blotches. Used topically, hydroquinone removes abnormally pigmented areas of skin and evens out skin color. Dermatologists typically recommend a 4 percent hydroquinone formulation. It is usually applied twice a day, or as directed by your physician.

The research is clear: When your skin-care program incorporates AHAs, expect to see dramatic improvements in fine lines (particularly around the eyes), leathery skin, discoloration, skin tone, and overall quality.

Moisturize the Skin

In the strictest sense AHAs and BHAs are not true moisturizers but have the rather amazing ability to draw moisture from the lower levels of the skin to promote suppleness. Thus, when applied topically, they plump up the water content of the epidermis, moisturizing and softening the skin. The moisturizing properties of these acids smooth out fine lines and help your skin maintain its natural supply of water.

WHICH HYDROXY ACID IS BEST?

Most hydroxy acid preparations on the market contain either glycolic acid or lactic acid. Others preparations are formulated with mandelic acid (derived from bitter almonds), malic acid, tartaric acid, and citric acid. There is also the BHA, salicylic acid.

Is one better than another?

You can't go wrong using a glycolic or lactic acid–based product. Both AHAs have been heavily researched for their antiaging and antiwrinkle benefits. Glycolic acid, in particular, has the smallest molecular size of any AHA, meaning that it can better penetrate the epidermal (topmost) layer of the skin. Glycolic acid and lactic acid stimulate skin-cell turnover and renewal at roughly equal rates when applied in the same concentrations and at the same pH.

Mandelic acid, on the other hand, has not been as well researched as a skin rejuvenator and is used in only a few cosmetics. Nor has tartaric acid been well scrutinized; however, among AHAs, it is one of the better performers when it comes to moisturizing the skin. As for malic acid, it doesn't have as much research behind it, either. One study found that when human-skin fibroblasts, isolated in lab dishes, were treated with either malic acid or glycolic acid, only glycolic acid increased the production of collagen.

Citric acid looks promising, though. In a study published in 1997, volunteers applied citric acid (a 20 percent solution with a 3.5 pH) twice a day to sun-damaged skin on one of their forearms and a placebo lotion to the other forearm. After three months of application, topical citric acid increased the thickness of the epidermis. There was also an increase in the GAG content in the dermis. The authors of this study noted that the skin changes produced by citric acid are similar to those observed with treatment by glycolic acid, lactic acid, and even tretinoin.

Though not as well studied as glycolic acid or lactic acid, salicylic acid has three attributes that make it a worthy contender for fighting age-related skin changes. First, it exfoliates at a deeper level than AHAs do. Second, it's less irritating to the skin, making it a good choice for women with sensitive skin. And third, as an aspirin spin-off, it reduces skin inflammation brought on by sun exposure. Among the products containing salicylic acid is Oil of Olay Daily Renewal Cream. It is formulated with 1.5 percent salicylic acid in a moisturizing cream base.

Numerous products contain mixtures of different types of acids. Combination products like these haven't been well tested. Nonetheless, if you opt for this type of product, buy it from well-known manufacturers.

HOW LONG WILL IT TAKE TO SEE RESULTS?

Within two to three weeks of regular use, your skin should begin to feel softer and exhibit a more rosy glow. Based on scientific research with hydroxy acids, it may take several additional months before fine lines, wrinkles, and other imperfections begin to diminish. With ongoing usage, the overall appearance, integrity, and quality of your skin will continue to improve.

How Do AHAs and BHAs Compare to Retinoids Such As Renova or Retin-A?

Quite probably, if you took a consensus of dermatologists, they would say that tretinoin (Renova or Retin-A) outperforms hydroxy acids when it comes to reducing wrinkles. (The retinoid, retinol, however, is thought to be equal in strength to AHAs.)

In truth, few adequate studies have been done comparing the AHAs with tretinoin. Writing in *Postgraduate Medicine,* renowned dermatologist Alfred M. Kligman, M.D., Ph.D., noted: "No other known chemicals or drugs can duplicate the diversity of anatomic and physiologic effects brought about by retinoids."

Still, many physicians prescribe skin-care regimens of tretinoin and AHAs together as a one-two punch against wrinkles and photodamage. Combining the two seems logical to get the best of both worlds, but studies are needed to verify the benefits of AHAs and tretinoin used in this way.

Are Hydroxy Acids Safe?

In rare cases, hydroxy acids have been known to cause redness, rash, itching, swelling (particularly around the eye area), burning, blistering, or bleeding. Since 1989, the Food and Drug Administration (FDA) has received 100 complaints on AHAs from consumers who have experienced one or more of these side effects. The FDA believes, however, that adverse reactions may be more widespread. In fact, the agency estimates that for every complaint it receives, a single manufacturer receives 50 to 100. As a result, the FDA is eyeing AHAs and their related compounds very carefully, particularly for their long-term effects, which are currently unknown.

Even so, AHAs and their relatives got a thumbs-up in 1997 by the Cosmetic Ingredient Review Panel—the cosmetic industry's own watchdog group for assessing the safety of cosmetic ingredients. After a two-year review, the panel concluded that these compounds are safe for over-the-counter consumer use when:

◊ The concentration is 10 percent or less.

◊ The product has a pH of 3.5 or higher.

◊ The product is formulated to protect the skin from sun, or contains label warnings advising consumers to practice daily sun protection.

For AHA products intended for salon use, the panel stated that formulations of glycolic acid and lactic acid at concentrations of 30 percent or less and a pH of 3 or higher should be intended for brief, onetime use, followed by thorough rinsing and regular use of sunscreen.

Some research indicates that using AHAs may make your skin overly sensitive to sunlight, especially if you have light hair and fair skin. But these findings have been disputed, primarily because a couple of studies indicate that topical glycolic acid, in particular, protects the skin against sun damage. Further, one study found that daily treatment of sunburned skin with glycolic acid accelerated healing. Without a doubt, more research is needed on this issue to see how it all shakes out.

So unless your skin is highly sensitive, hydroxy acids have virtually no side effects, particularly when used as directed. Although the product may feel irritating at first, this initial irritation will subside with time. Should you have an adverse reaction, however, stop using the product and consult a dermatologist.

GUIDELINES FOR APPLYING HYDROXY ACIDS

With any hydroxy acid product, follow the manufacturer's instructions for application. Most AHAs or BHAs are designed to be applied once or twice a day. You can continue to use them indefinitely, or for as long as you desire to improve the appearance of your skin.

In addition, you can use them with your regular cosmetics and sunscreens. In fact, your foundation will go on more easily and uniformly, particularly after you've used a hydroxy acid product for at least two to three weeks. This is because the exfoliating and moisturizing actions of hydroxy acids, when they are used consistently, smooth out the skin.

Here are some additional guidelines for the safe use of AHAs and BHAs:

◊ Apply a sunscreen (SPF 15 or higher) to your skin before going out, and wear sun-protective clothing.

◊ Read the labels to identify which hydroxy acid and other chemicals are present in the product. It is optional for manufacturers to list the hydroxy concentration and pH level on the label or in their product literature. However, you should be able to write or call the manufacturer to obtain this information.

◊ Test the product on a small patch of skin if you have never used hydroxy acids before or if you are switching to a more concentrated product.

◊ To minimize irritation, wash your hands prior to applying the product and apply the product sparingly.

◊ Stop using the product if you experience untoward reactions such as redness, itching, burning, pain, bleeding, or increased sensitivity to sunlight. Consult your dermatologist to rule out other possible causes for the adverse reaction.

PART FOUR

Natural Skin-Savers

7

The Skin Antioxidants

YOUR skin is not only a functioning organ but also an elaborate defense system against hostile surroundings. In fact, very few organs in the body are subjected to as many environmental assaults as your skin. Sunlight, ozone, air pollutants, chemical toxins, invasions by microorganisms, burns, and wounds are just a few of the offenders.

When skin is exposed to an offending agent—particularly ultraviolet radiation—free radicals are generated. As explained earlier, free radicals contain one or more unpaired and unstable electrons. Highly reactive, free radicals roam the body unchecked, grabbing electrons of other molecules and claiming them as their own. The process of pairing up with molecules for electrons is called *cellular oxidation.* Cellular oxidation is similar to the reaction that rusts metal or turns oils rancid, and it's just as damaging to the body.

In your skin, oxidative damage can occur in three major sites: the fatty layers of cell membranes, in DNA (the genetic material inside cells), and in proteins. In a domino-like series of chemical reactions, free radicals hook up with fatty acids in cell membranes to form substances called *peroxides*. Peroxides attack cell membranes, setting off a chain reaction that creates many more free radicals. Pits form in cell membranes, allowing harmful bacteria, viruses, and other disease-causing agents to gain entry into cells. Technically, this process is known as *lipid peroxidation*.

In addition, free radicals can actually break or alter DNA, potentially leading to various disorders, including premature aging and cancer. Further, free radicals are responsible for degrading collagen, elastin, and other proteins in the skin.

A key line of defense against these attacks involves specialized nutrients called antioxidants. Vitamin C, vitamin E, and beta-carotene are the chief vitamin antioxidants. They work in various ways to arrest free radicals.

Among the antioxidant minerals are zinc, selenium, and copper. They supply the elements your body needs to make *antioxidant enzymes*. In general, enzymes are proteins that bring about chemical changes inside cells; antioxidant enzymes inactivate free radicals. Glutathione peroxidase, for example, is an antioxidant enzyme produced by selenium with the power to turn troublesome free radicals into harmless water. Copper and zinc help make superoxide dismutase (SOD), an antioxidant enzyme that inactivates certain free radicals.

Hundreds of face creams, marketed as antiaging products, are formulated with antioxidants. The most commonly used antioxidants in these products are vitamin C, vitamin E, and coenzyme Q10, although many other antioxidants are being evaluated for potential use against skin aging. Here's a closer look at skin antioxidants and how they work.

VITAMIN C

When you read about vitamin C, it is usually in reference to its cold-fighting power. But did you know that vitamin C—the most commonly supplemented nutrient in the United States—can also help erase fine wrinkles and firm up skin when applied topically?

That's right. Vitamin C, also known as ascorbic acid, is an antioxidant that keeps free radicals from destroying the outermost layers of cells. It also has the power to regenerate vitamin E, another antioxidant. Because of its antioxidant properties, topical vitamin C is a potent weapon against sun-induced skin aging. It is particularly effective for fighting wrinkles, reducing freckles, softening leathery skin, and restoring the elasticity of skin.

Vitamin C is one of the "water-soluble" vitamins. This means that it is picked up by body fluids, transported by the bloodstream, and excreted in urine. Because our bodies cannot manufacture vitamin C, we must procure it from our diets or through supplementation. Foods rich in vitamin C include citrus fruits, green and red peppers, collard greens, broccoli, brussels sprouts, cabbage, spinach, potatoes, cantaloupe, and strawberries.

Of all the dietary vitamin C absorbed by our bodies, only about 8 percent is taken up by the skin. As a water-soluble nutrient, vitamin C is not easily stored. In fact, it remains in the body less than 20 days and must be replenished. Even then, its antioxidant activity can be crippled by ultraviolet-A (UVA) radiation. When your skin is deprived of antioxidants, including vitamin C, there is increased destruction of collagen and elastin, and photoaging speeds up. Nourishing your skin with topical vitamin C prevents many of the disastrous effects of photoaging.

How Does Topical Vitamin C Work?

Found in serums, creams, and lotions, vitamin C confers
some rather amazing benefits. For example, vitamin C:

Protects Against the Harmful Effects of Sunlight

Ultraviolet radiation stimulates the formation of free radicals, which in turn mutate cells and destroy collagen,
elastin, and other structures that give skin its youthful
firmness and elasticity. But by increasing the concentration
of vitamin C in skin, you can potentially protect skin cells
from this degree of damage. That's the finding of a 1992
study conducted at Duke University Medical Center,
where scientists examined the effects of multiple applications of topical vitamin C on the skin of pigs who were exposed to sunlight.

The scientists discovered that vitamin C prevented redness, plus reduced the formation and number of sunburned
cells. They attributed these benefits to vitamin C's ability
to counteract free radicals generated by ultraviolet radiation. Equally impressive: Topical vitamin C remained protective for up to three days.

Worth clarifying is that topical vitamin C does not block
or absorb harmful ultraviolet rays like sunscreen does. Instead, it neutralizes skin-damaging free radicals and thus
protects skin from photoaging. Also, unlike sunscreen, topical vitamin C becomes incorporated into the skin and will
not wash off with bathing, wiping, or exercising.

Reduces Inflammation Associated with Sunburn

Inflammation is the body's natural reaction to any type of
injury, including sunburn. Inflamed tissues become red,

swollen, and often painful. Inflammation sets off the production of free radicals.

Vitamin C acts as a natural anti-inflammatory. In a small study with human volunteers exposed to inflammation-producing agents, sites pretreated with vitamin C (a 10 percent concentration) showed a 22 percent reduction in inflammation.

Boosts Collagen Production

One of vitamin C's most important tasks is to produce and maintain collagen in organs and tissues throughout the body, including skin. Scientists have directly observed this production process in the lab. In a couple of studies, collagen production was stimulated after vitamin C was introduced into the fibroblasts of human skin. Fibroblasts are the cells that give rise to new collagen and elastin. Of course more studies like this are needed, but these observations are exciting, nonetheless.

Heals Skin Irritation Following Laser Resurfacing

Laser resurfacing is a procedure performed by a plastic surgeon or a dermatologic surgeon. Using a special laser beam, the surgeon removes photodamaged areas of the epidermis. The goal of laser resurfacing is to minimize and reduce deep wrinkles. A side effect of the procedure is skin irritation and inflammation. When applied about two weeks after the procedure, topical vitamin C decreases these side effects and cuts healing time nearly in half. Topical vitamin C is also recommended for use following a chemical face peel.

NOURISHING YOUR SKIN WITH
TOPICAL VITAMIN C

Nearly all major cosmetics companies market skin-care
products formulated with vitamin C. Some examples in-
clude Vitabolic, a gel cream manufactured by Lancôme
(L'Oréal); Synergie C, a moisturizer also from L'Oréal;
Clearly C 10% Vitamin C Serum from Avon; and Visible
Difference Pore-fix C, a cleansing system from Elizabeth
Arden.

One of the better-known topical vitamin C products is
Cellex-C. It was developed in the eighties by a cell biolo-
gist named Lorraine Meisner from the University of Wisconsin, Madison. Meisner, in fact, was the first
investigator to theorize that vitamin C, when applied topically and directly to the skin, could reverse sagging and
wrinkling.

A problem with vitamin C at the time was that it was
very unstable and could not easily penetrate the skin.
Working in the kitchen of her home, Meisner experi-
mented and devised a mixture of 10 percent ascorbic acid
with the mineral zinc and the amino acid tyrosine. The
mixture proved stable and absorbable by the skin. She
tested her formulation in clinical trials and received a
patent for it in 1990. Celeel Hayden LLC bought the right
to manufacture it, and since then, the product has become
a huge success. Cellex-C also contains some botanicals,
which are believed to promote skin elasticity.

Regular use of Cellex-C appears to rejuvenate the skin.
A recent clinical trial of Cellex-C attests to this benefit. For
three months, 19 patients (ages 36 to 72) with mild to moderate photodamage applied three drops of Cellex-C serum to
one side of the face and three drops of a placebo serum to the
other side. The patients did not know which serum contained the active agent, topical ascorbic acid.

For comparative purposes, photographs and computerized images of the patients' faces were taken prior to the start of the study. By the end of the experimental period, wrinkling, surface roughness, yellowness, looseness, and other skin irregularities had improved significantly in the skin treated with Cellex-C.

Put another way: In only three months, your skin may appear firmer and smoother, plus show visibly improved texture and color, with the use of a natural, nonprescription product. These are certainly encouraging findings.

You can purchase Cellex-C through professional aestheticians, dermatologists, plastic surgeons, or through the Web site, www.cellex-c.com. No prescription is required. A stronger formulation (Advanced-C Serum) containing 17.5 percent ascorbic acid is available, too. If you use Cellex-C, it should be applied to a clean, dry face, once every 24 hours.

Most topical vitamin C products are formulated with ascorbic acid, which is water soluble; some contain ascorbyl palmitate, a synthetic ester of vitamin C that is fat soluble. ("Fat soluble" means that it can be stored with fat in the liver and other tissues.) Referred to as *vitamin C ester,* ascorbyl palmitate is rapidly absorbed by the skin by virtue of its fat solubility. Research shows that it is a powerful anti-inflammatory agent that can prevent free-radical damage. Vitamin C ester also stimulates the growth of skin fibroblasts in lab dishes. A line of products formulated with this form of vitamin C is the Vitamin C Ester Collection, available at many major department stores and through the Web site www.nvperriconemd.com.

Topical vitamin C products appear to have no side effects. They can be used on virtually all skin types.

VITAMIN E

Another powerful skin antioxidant is vitamin E, a fat-soluble vitamin. Technically, vitamin E is known as *tocopherol,* a term derived from a Greek word meaning "offspring." It was given this name more than 75 years ago when researchers discovered a substance in vegetable oils that was necessary for reproduction in rats. That substance later came to be known as vitamin E. Over time, four different tocopherols were identified and differentiated by one of the first four letters of the Greek alphabet: alpha, beta, gamma, and delta. The most biologically active of the four is alpha tocopherol.

Vitamin E is distributed widely in foods, and the richest sources are vegetable oils and products made from them. Wheat germ and nuts are high in vitamin E, too, and fruits and vegetables supply appreciable amounts.

Vitamin E is a component of cells, sandwiched between the fatty layers that make up cell membranes. When free radicals come along, they hitch up to vitamin E, damaging it instead of the rest of the cell membrane. In the process, vitamin E soaks up the free radicals, and the cell is protected from damage. Vitamin C and other antioxidants can regenerate vitamin E. But with a shortage of vitamin E, there's an increase in free radicals, cellular injuries, and subsequent disorders to bodily tissues, including accelerated aging of the skin.

As a skin antioxidant, topical vitamin E has been getting its share of the antiaging spotlight and may someday rival vitamin C as a natural and very potent wrinkle-fighter. It is not yet as well researched as topical vitamin C, however. Also, vitamin E does not penetrate the skin very well, unless formulated in special water-based lotions or creams. Nonetheless, dermatologists and skin researchers feel that vitamin E holds great promise in treating skin conditions. For example, vitamin E:

May Minimize Wrinkles

Vitamin E is proving its worth as a wrinkle-fighter. In one study involving hairless mice, topical vitamin E reduced the severity of skin wrinkling by a whopping 75 percent! (Hairless mice are used frequently in dermatologic experiments because their skin ages and reacts to sunlight in the same manner as human skin does, only in a shorter time period.)

Experiments with mice are one thing, but what about humans? Does topical vitamin E work the same wonders? Already, some preliminary research says—yes. In one study, investigators tested a 5 percent solution of natural vitamin E in a cream base that was applied to the outer eye areas of volunteers. The study lasted four weeks. Compared with the placebo, the vitamin E cream visibly reduced the depth of wrinkles, the length of facial lines, and the surface roughness of skin. These findings are encouraging news, particularly if you have crow's-feet.

Protects Collagen

Whereas topical vitamin C stimulates the production of skin-firming collagen, topical vitamin E protects it from destruction. In a Japanese study published in 1993, investigators observed that vitamin E completely prevented free radicals from injuring collagen in human-skin fibroblasts, isolated in lab dishes.

More recently, a group of French scientists discovered that vitamin E interfered with the activity of collagen-destroying enzymes in human skin. This body of research hints that topical vitamin E could be the next big thing when it comes to preventing wrinkles.

Guards Against Sunburn

The reason you find vitamin E in so many sunscreen products is that it protects skin against the harmful effects of ultraviolet radiation. This benefit has been proved in both animal and human studies.

Further, scientists at the North Carolina Biotechnology Center in Raleigh found that a combination of vitamin C and vitamin E, formulated with a commercial sunscreen (oxybenzone), provided superior protection against photodamage. Other research shows that both topical antioxidants work best when applied prior to going out in the sun.

The mechanism by which vitamin E protects against sunburn is unclear, however. But because vitamin E cannot absorb enough ultraviolet radiation to fully shield the skin, scientists speculate that its antioxidant action is the force behind its powerful protection.

Works As an Anti-Inflammatory Agent

In animal studies, topical vitamin E significantly reduced the redness and swelling (both symptoms of inflammation) caused by exposure to ultraviolet light. When inflammation is diminished, free radicals are less likely to do their dirty work.

Softens the Skin

Incorporated into moisturizers and other creams or lotions, vitamin E helps soften, smooth, and moisturize the skin. Researchers found that when 20 women applied an 8 percent vitamin E cream to their skin for 10 days, the smoothness of their skin was enhanced considerably, even after it had been purposely exposed to artificial ultraviolet light on three occasions during the experiment.

In a study published in 1998, German scientists found

that a 5 percent concentration of vitamin E in an emulsion significantly increased water content in the stratum corneum, the visible outer layer of the epidermis. In essence, vitamin E helped moisturize the skin by keeping it well hydrated. Many skin specialists feel that properly moisturizing the skin can slow down or minimize the effects of aging.

BETA-CAROTENE

Beta-carotene is a member of a group of substances known as *carotenoids*. There are more than 600 carotenoids in nature, found mostly in orange and yellow fruits and vegetables and dark green vegetables. Beta-carotene was the first carotenoid to be isolated and is the most widely studied.

Once ingested, beta-carotene is converted to vitamin A (retinol) in the body on an as-needed basis. As an antioxidant, beta-carotene's main role is to detoxify a highly energetic, free-radical-like product called *singlet oxygen*. Sunlight-induced singlet oxygen mutates DNA in skin fibroblasts, a process that accelerates extrinsic aging in human skin.

Clinically, though, it's not yet clear how beta-carotene may directly slow down or reverse skin aging. However, the nutrient is used for treating photosensitive disorders— conditions in which the skin is abnormally sensitive to light. Left untreated, photosensitivity leads to severe sunburn, hives, swelling or blistering of the skin, or other serious health problems. In a study of patients with a photosensitive disorder, supplemental beta-carotene significantly increased their tolerance to sunlight.

Apparently, the nutrient can do the same for healthy individuals. Research shows that by supplementing with oral beta-carotene, you may be able to stay out in the sun a little longer before getting sunburned. It is generally recommended that you take beta-carotene supplements over a four-to-six-week period prior to increased sun exposure because it takes several weeks for the nutrient to build up in the skin. Scientists believe that beta-carotene works by causing slight changes in skin pigmentation and preventing free-radical damage to the skin.

Taking beta-carotene and using sunscreen affords even greater protection. So does supplementing with vitamin E. Researchers found that a carotenoid supplement (25 milligrams) and a vitamin E supplement (500 IU) taken daily for 12 weeks diminished sunburn (induced by a solar simulator) in 20 volunteers far more than a supplement of carotenoids alone.

Beta-carotene has not been employed much as a topical agent, except in animal studies, where it has been tested primarily as a treatment for oral cancer. Instead, beta-carotene exerts its sun protection *systemically*. This means that when consumed in food or supplements, beta-carotene enters the bloodstream and is delivered to tissues and organs to do its work.

For an extra measure of protection, you may want to take supplemental beta-carotene. For general health, a daily dosage of 25,000 IU (15 milligrams) is reasonable. If you exceed that dosage, say 30 milligrams or more a day for a long period of time, your skin may turn yellow because beta-carotene accumulates in the fat layer underneath the dermis. Stop oversupplementing and this condition will disappear.

COENZYME Q10

Technically known as *ubiquinone,* coenzyme Q10 (abbreviated as coQ10) is a nutrient found naturally inside cells, where it is involved in the conversion of food to energy. It also acts as an antioxidant capable of disarming free radicals. The skin contains high levels of coQ10.

As an oral supplement, coQ10 has many health-giving properties. For example, it helps improve cardiac function, strengthens the immune system, and may enhance the quality of overall health.

Now a topical form of coQ10 is gaining notoriety as a wrinkle-stopper. With age, your body produces less coQ10 and, consequently, there is less of its antioxidant power to go around. This is bad news for skin cells because, in theory, low levels of coQ10 can show up as skin aging. By replenishing your skin with coQ10, though, you can potentially fend off or reverse wrinkles and other signs of skin aging.

Skin creams formulated with coQ10 are designed to counter photoaging—including wrinkles—which takes place over time from long-term exposure of the skin to the sun.

A recent study with 20 volunteers found that a 0.3 percent coQ10 cream (Nivea Visage Q10 Wrinkle Control Crème) has the power to prevent the many of the effects of photodamage. Applied once daily to the skin around the eyes, the cream reduced wrinkle depth, suppressed free-radical damage, and interfered with the destructive action of collagenase, one of the enzymes that break down collagen. The study lasted six months, but now Nivea asserts that the product can reduce wrinkles in just 10 weeks. These findings are certainly good news for anyone with prematurely aged skin—and crow's-feet.

It is worth mentioning, too, that excessive exposure to ultraviolet radiation can rapidly deplete levels of coQ10 in the skin. Because a study with rats found that coQ10 can easily penetrate the skin, scientists believe that topical formulations of this antioxidant may help protect the skin against excessive sunlight—in addition to its antiwrinkle benefits. CoQ10 is found in an increasing number of skin creams.

Alpha Lipoic Acid

On the antiwrinkle center stage of late is alpha lipoic acid, a vitaminlike nutrient made naturally in the body and available from foods such as potatoes and red meat. One of its main talents is as an antioxidant to protect the body against mischief-making free radicals. As explained above, your body has a whole brigade of free-radical terminators that include vitamin C, vitamin E, and beta-carotene. In the process of terminating free radicals, however, these antioxidants are often temporarily wounded. Happily, though, they can be regenerated to their original form by other antioxidants. Alpha lipoic acid is one of the chief antioxidants with the power to do this. In essence, it preserves and boosts the level of antioxidants in the skin, shoring up defenses against aging.

Alpha lipoic acid has other protective talents. Free radicals activate a cellular messenger that enters the nucleus of cells and forces DNA to produce proteins that cause cellular damage. Alpha lipoic acid, along with other antioxidants, can put the brakes on this process in order to protect cells. It terminates a free radical known as the *hydroxyl radical,* which happens to be the most damaging to the body.

Alpha lipoic acid also helps manufacture glutathione, a protein produced in the liver. Glutathione itself is a powerful antioxidant that guards the body against ultraviolet radiation, cigarette smoke, and other environmental toxins that can accelerate skin aging. It is also a constituent of glutathione peroxidase, an important member of the antioxidant enzyme defense team in the skin.

Alpha lipoic acid is now available topically in skin-care cosmetics such as Face Firming Activator with NTP Complex, sold in some department stores and from the Web site www.nvperriconemd.com. Because it is both water and fat soluble, topical alpha lipoic acid penetrates the skin rapidly and easily makes its way into cells.

As a treatment for aging skin, topical alpha lipoic acid has been found to diminish fine lines within only a few weeks, prevent sunburn, and work as an anti-inflammatory to soothe the skin. It has also demonstrated the ability to minimize acne scarring with six to eight weeks of continual use.

Topical alpha lipoic acid is appropriate for all skin types. So promising is this antioxidant as a natural treatment for wrinkles that I believe we will hear much more about it in the future.

OTHER SKIN-PROTECTING ANTIOXIDANTS

Other skin antioxidants that deserve mention are the minerals copper, zinc, and selenium. Copper is involved in making collagen and elastin and aids in the production of GAGs. It also helps synthesize superoxide dismutase (SOD), an antioxidant enzyme that is very active in the skin. Because of these roles, copper may be an important topical nutrient for the skin. Copper peptides (a copper/protein combination) are the chief ingredients in a line of skin-care products from ProCyte Corporation called the Neova Therapies. For information on these products, access the company's Web site at www.procyte.com.

Zinc is an ingredient of some topical products, including Cellex-C. Present in every nook and cranny of the body, zinc has an array of functions. Among the most important is promoting the general growth of all body tissues, including skin and hair. Zinc is also involved in manufacturing collagen.

When added to cultured human-skin fibroblasts that had been zapped with ultraviolet-A radiation, zinc prevented DNA from breaking and delayed cell death, according to a 1999 study conducted in France. Zinc has also been shown to reduce lipid peroxidation in human-skin fibroblasts that have been exposed to ultraviolet radiation.

Studies of skin cells, isolated in lab dishes, indicate that selenium also helps protect skin fibroblasts from ultraviolet damage. What's more, it appears to preserve the elasticity of the skin by delaying the oxidation of fatty acids when taken orally.

WHEN TO APPLY TOPICAL ANTIOXIDANTS

Topical antioxidants are often used in partnership with other skin-rejuvenating cosmetics such as Renova or hydroxy acids. That way, your skin gets the best combination of antiaging care. In fact, many dermatologists are now advising the use of a "system" of skin-care products.

How, then, do you incorporate topical antioxidants into a total skin-care system?

Renova and Retin-A are always applied at night because their active ingredient, tretinoin, is degraded by sunlight. So in the morning, after cleansing your face, apply your topical antioxidant, followed by sunscreen. If you don't use Renova or Retin-A, apply your hydroxy acid product in the evening before going to bed.

Because topical vitamin C, tretinoin, and hydroxy acids can dry and possibly inflame your skin, it's probably not a good idea to use all three every day. You might consider rotating their use: tretinoin on Monday, Wednesday, and Friday; topical vitamin C or hydroxy acids on the other days. But first, discuss this regimen with your dermatologist.

Some topical antioxidants are designed for nightly use only. One example is Avon's Formula C Patches, which are applied to trouble spots such as crow's-feet and laugh lines, and kept there while you sleep. No matter which product you use, always follow the manufacturer's directions for application.

8
Return-to-Youth Botanicals

A natural approach to antiaging has been taking hold in the cosmetics industry as more companies formulate products with plant-based ingredients designed to smooth out wrinkles and restore the look of youth. Skin-care products containing *botanicals* (herbs or constituents of herbs) are believed to be gentler on the skin than substances such as tretinoin or hydroxy acids.

But the question is: Do such products actually work?

Research on antiwrinkle botanicals hasn't quite caught up to the volumes of information we have on tretinoin, hydroxy acids, or topical vitamins. Nonetheless, there are some promising new developments in topical botanicals that are of interest if you're gravitating toward natural treatments for wrinkles.

KINERASE

A hormone that makes plants grow and thrive is one of the latest skin-savers to hit the antiaging market. That hormone is N6-furfuryladenine—a naturally occurring growth factor in plants that prevents the aging of leaves and keeps them moist. It is the active ingredient in Kinerase, a skincare product launched to U.S. consumers in 1999. Kinerase is available as a cream or lotion, formulated with a 0.1 percent concentration of N6-furfuryladenine.

The antiaging benefits of N6-furfuryladenine were first reported in 1994 by researchers in Denmark who examined its effects on human-skin fibroblasts. Their studies found that N6-furfuryladenine improved skin roughness, fine wrinkling, and blotchiness.

In clinical trials conducted by a dermatology department at the University of California, Irvine, Kinerase significantly reversed the signs of photodamage in patients who used the product for 24 weeks. It reduced the appearance of wrinkles, minimized age spots, and prevented moisture loss, all while improving skin texture. ICN Pharmaceuticals, which manufactures Kinerase, says you should begin to see results in four to six weeks.

N6-furfuryladenine is a known antioxidant as well, with the ability to hunt down and destroy free radicals. Unlike some antiwrinkle agents, it is not an exfoliant and will not promote the shedding of dead skin cells.

Kathy A. Fields, M.D., a leading dermatologist, had this to say about Kinerase in an article she wrote for the *International Journal of Fertility and Women's Medicine:* "My personal experience with Kinerase has been fairly good. It is certainly not a 'face-lift in a jar,' as none of these [topical antioxidants] are; however, the texture of patients' skin has been found to improve, pigment has also improved modestly with good sun protection, and fine wrinkling has improved modestly, particularly under the eyes, and very slightly around the lips."

Using Kinerase

Kinerase is applied to sun-damaged areas of the body—face, neck, shoulders, chest, or hands—once or twice a day. You can use it with makeup and sunscreen. Kinerase is suitable for all skin types, and it does not cause allergies, acne, or blemishes. Nor does it make your skin sensitive to sunlight. In fact, Kinerase has virtually no side effects and will not burn, sting, peel, or otherwise irritate your skin.

Kinerase is available from dermatologists and plastic surgeons, but without a prescription. You can find out more about the product by calling 1-877-KINERASE or accessing the product's Web site at www.kinerase.com.

PROCYANIDINS

Procyanidins are a group of natural chemicals found most abundantly in grape seeds and in the bark of the French maritime pine, which grows along the coast of southern France. Also known as procyanidolic ogliomers or OPCs, procyanidins are used increasingly in skin-care products because they are powerful antioxidants. In fact, research shows that their antioxidant activity is 50 times more potent than vitamin E and 20 times greater than vitamin C. What's more, they protect vitamin E and vitamin C in the skin from being overwhelmed by free radicals. And because procyanidins have a small molecular structure, they are well absorbed by the skin.

Processed from the pits of grapes, grape-seed extract is found in Vinefit from Lancôme, a vitamin-enriched moisturizer. French maritime pine-bark extract contains a procyanidin called *pycnogenol,* which is found in numerous wrinkle creams, including Correct from ZIRH Skin Nutrition.

Topically applied products containing procyanidins positively influence the appearance of skin in several ways. For example, procyanidins:

Help Strengthen Tissue

Maintaining the structural integrity of the underlying skin is key to reducing wrinkles. Procyanidins preserve connective tissue by interfering with the activity of destructive enzymes that break down collagen, elastin, and hyaluronic acid (a natural lubricant in skin). In animal research, investigators demonstrated that procyanidins can attach themselves to elastin fibers in skin and protect these fibers from breakdown by elastin-destroying enzymes. In addition, procyanidins may actually help rebuild collagen in the skin for a smoother, firmer appearance.

Protect Against UVB Rays

Known as the "sunburn radiation," UVB light penetrates the epidermis and cripples your skin's natural antioxidant defense system, rendering it virtually powerless against skin-damaging free radicals. Studies hint that pycnogenol, in particular, reduces skin-cell damage caused by UVB radiation and scavenges the free radicals it generates. Pycnogenol is also an anti-inflammatory agent. Whenever skin inflammation can be reduced, free radicals stay in check.

Improve Circulation

Often used in the treatment of circulatory disorders, procyanidins improve blood and oxygen flow by dilating blood vessels. They also protect capillary walls and promote normal permeability of capillaries. Both actions have a normalizing effect on surrounding tissues. When circulation is enhanced, skin cells are better nourished. The removal of toxins and waste products from the dermis and epidermis speeds up, too.

Poor skin circulation can lead to water retention, a condition that puffs up the skin around your eyelids. Using topically applied pycnogenol may help reduce this sort of puffiness.

Procyanidin Products

Cosmetics formulated with procyanidins will say so on the label. Look for such designations as grape-seed polyphenol, grape-seed extract, pycnogenol, or bioflavonoids.

LEMON OIL

From that lemon you squeeze into your tea or on your fish comes an oily extract that reduces free-radical damage to the skin and may help reverse skin aging. In 1999, researchers in Italy isolated a new compound from lemon oil—they dubbed it Lem1—that appears to protect the skin from the onslaught of free radicals.

In their study, they set out to learn how the lemon oil extract compared with vitamin E in terms of reducing lipid peroxidation—the destruction of cell membranes that is generated by free radicals. The researchers recruited 30 adult men (ages 28 to 44) and instructed one group of men to apply vitamin E to their forehead and another group to apply Lem1 to their forehead as well. As a control, skin surface lipids were taken from the forehead of each subject. The study lasted one week. Three times during that period, researchers examined skin lipid samples taken by swabbing the subjects' foreheads. The extracted samples were exposed to chemicals that induced free-radical activity.

What the researchers discovered was intriguing: The lemon oil extract boosted antioxidant activity in the skin significantly—even better than vitamin E did. Further, the protective effect of Lem1 was evident from the first day of treatment and remained effective throughout the experimental period. The researchers noted: "These experiments clearly indicate that Lem1 is endowed with considerably high antioxidant activity."

Because free-radical damage is one of the chief causes of skin aging, lemon oil extract may represent a natural yet very potent way to fight wrinkles. Hopefully, more research will be conducted on lemon oil to verify the positive findings discovered thus far.

AYURVEDA SKIN CARE

From the oldest of all medicinal systems, Ayurveda (pronounced eye-yuhr-VAY-dah), comes one of the newest ways to potentially reduce wrinkles. Used for more than 5,000 years in India, Ayurveda treats diseases holistically, with nutrition, exercise, meditation, and other lifestyle-management approaches.

Ayurveda classifies individuals into three health/body types, governed by controlling principles called *Vata, Pitta,* or *Kapha.* According to Ayurvedic thought, all three intermingle in an individual's constitution, to some degree, although a single principle may predominate or be out of balance at any given time. You're considered healthy if all three principles are in equilibrium.

Practitioners look at the patient's disposition, habits, and life in general in order to customize the Ayurvedic treatment. Integral to healing is the use of more than 2,000 therapeutic herbs, many of which are native to India. Most are taken orally, while others are applied topically to treat skin diseases.

So popular is this system of natural health that many companies have introduced Ayurvedic cosmetics. One of the newest is the Youthful Skin Line from MAPI, developed by Dr. Rama Kant Mishra, an Ayurvedic dermatologist. Designed for women ages 35 to 55, it features six topical products and an oral herbal supplement.

There are three main Ayurvedic herbs in these products. One of the most important is gotu kola, a member of the parsley family usually found growing in drainage ditches in Asia and orchards in Hawaii. A known effect of this herb is that it strengthens collagen to help improve the underlying integrity of the skin. What's more, the herb may regenerate collagen and protect it from sun-induced damage.

The other two herbs found in these cosmetics are sensitive plant (mimosa), which acts as an astringent and reduces swelling, and flame of forest, which protects against UV radiation.

The company's Youth Skin Cream, which also contains alpha hydroxy acids, was tested on 20 women by an independent lab. The experiment found that the cream, applied twice a day, improved skin thickness by 14 percent and reduced fine lines by 39 percent. In addition, the cream enhanced skin moisture, firmness and smoothness. The first signs of improvement became apparent after a month of use, with continued progress after 12 weeks of use. For more information on the Youthful Skin line, access the Web site www.maharishiAyurveda.com.

Other herbs believed to be therapeutic in Ayurvedic skin care are pongamia extract, shown to absorb skin-damaging UVA rays; vitamin C-rich Indian gooseberry; guggul, a gum resin that is an effective antiseptic; and licorice root, which has anti-inflammatory properties.

USING BOTANICALS

There are countless botanicals used in cosmetics today. Table 8.1 lists some of the more popular, along with their possible benefits. In most cases, botanically based cosmetics are gentle enough to be used daily, but you should always follow the manufacturer's directions. Discuss with your dermatologist whether it is wise to apply botanicals at the same time as tretinoin, hydroxy acids, or other topical products, since using a combination of cosmetics may irritate your skin and produce undesirable results.

Table 8.1: Skin-Loving Botanicals: A Primer

Almond oil	Rich in antioxidants and found in many moisturizers.
Aloe vera	Soothes the skin, holds in moisture, and acts as an anti-inflammatory.
Banana flower	May decrease the appearance of fine lines and firm the skin.
Burdock	Treats eczema and other skin conditions.
Calendula	Treats inflammation.
Centella asiatica	May decrease the appearance of fine lines and firm the skin.
Chamomile	Acts as an anti-inflammatory.
Cocoa butter	Remoisturizes the skin.
Cucumber	Reduces puffiness, tightens pores, and refreshes the skin.
Elderflower	Reduces undereye puffiness. Soothes dry skin.
Ginkgo biloba	A good skin antioxidant.
Green tea	Reduces redness.
Hazelnut extract	Softens skin.
Horsechestnut	An antioxidant that may help fight wrinkles.
Horsetail	Contains the mineral silica, which has been found in research to reduce wrinkling when applied topically.
Ivy	Steps up circulation to the skin.

Lavender	Soothes the skin.
Licorice	Moisturizes the skin.
Macadamia nut oil	Softens skin.
Mulberry	Moisturizes the skin.
Olive oil	Believed to slow wrinkling and most recently was found in a clinical trial with mice to reverse sun damage; also a powerful antioxidant.
Rose	Has cleansing and moisturizing properties.
Rosemary	Identified by Japanese researchers as a promising antiwrinkle herb; stimulates circulation.
Sage	Believed to have antiwrinkle properties; smoothes the skin.
Sandalwood	Soothes the skin.
Silymarin	A natural chemical found in artichokes and the milk thistle plant that protects against UVB radiation-induced skin damage.
Sunflower	Promotes skin firmness and suppleness.
Thyme	Moisturizes the skin.
Yarrow	Helps firms saggy skin.
Yucca root	Works as a cleanser and moisturizer.

9

Young Skin Secrets from the Sea

WHEN Ponce de León set out to find the fountain of youth, he may have been sailing on it all along—the sea. The sea is teeming with natural ingredients that skin-care companies are harvesting for a host of antiaging cosmetics. Many of these products have been scientifically tested and shown to smooth out wrinkles, restore elasticity, and regenerate sun- and time-damaged skin.

These marine-based ingredients include various types of fish extracts. Among them are *polysaccharides,* derived from the cartilage of fish. Polysaccharides are basically strings of sugar molecules that occur naturally in the bodily structures of various marine animals.

Another popular fish extract is an oil called *squalene,* obtained from shark-liver extract (as well as from olive oil) and used to make squalane, a similar compound used widely in cosmetics, particularly moisturizers. Squalene is also a part of human sebum, a yellowish, oily secretion involved in naturally lubricating the skin.

Also widely used in antiwrinkle cosmetics are seaweed extracts. Technically, seaweeds are known as algae and classified into groups by color: red, brown, and green. Algae are plants, although they lack true roots, stems, and leaves. Because the marine environment in which they grow is saturated with nutrients, algae are a treasure trove of proteins, polysaccharides, vitamins, and antioxidants that serve a variety of functions, particularly when incorporated into cosmetics.

In addition, marine silts and sediments are highly valued for their rich mineral content and used in masks, cleansers, and other topical products.

What follows is a closer look at marine-based cosmetics that show promise as a natural approach to smoothing out existing wrinkles and promoting healthier skin.

VIVIDA

From Helsinki, Finland, comes a line of cosmetics named Vivida, which includes topical products and an oral supplement. Vivida products are formulated with a special mixture of polysaccharides. For a nonprescription product, Vivida has been fairly well studied as an alternative therapy for aging skin.

Initial studies were conducted in 1992, with intriguing results. In Helsinki, researchers tested the effects of the Vivida oral supplement on sun-damaged skin of women, aged 40 to 60 years old. A group of 15 women took 500 milligrams of Vivida daily for three months, while a second group of 15 women supplemented with a placebo.

In the Vivida-treated women, the thickness of the epidermis and the dermis increased after three months. What's more, skin elasticity was enhanced significantly. No such changes occurred in the placebo-takers. Nor were any side effects reported.

Also in 1992, the same researchers tested the effects of Vivida cream on sun- and age-damaged skin over a period of four months. The cream is formulated with a mixture of polysaccharides, vitamin A, and vitamin E.

Thirty women participated in this study. Twice a day they applied Vivida cream to one side of their face and a placebo cream to the other. The positive effects of the Vivida cream were apparent after just 28 days.

Again, Vivida outperformed the placebo, thickening the epidermis and the dermis. The cream also increased skin elasticity significantly and reduced the mottled appearance of the subjects' complexion. No side effects were reported.

An Italian study conducted on Vivida corroborated these findings. Researchers gave 30 women with sun-damaged skin two pills of Vivida daily or a placebo. After three months, those taking Vivida saw significant improvement in their skin structure, as well as diminished fine lines and deep wrinkles. There was no improvement observed in the placebo group.

The researchers wrote: "During discussions with the females who received the active treatment [Vivida], it became definitely clear that all of them were highly satisfied with the result of the treatment and that all of them would have liked to be on the same treatment for a longer period of time. The females in the placebo group were very impressed by the results in the activity treated group and wished to receive the active Vivida tablets."

How exactly do these natural marine proteins work to rejuvenate the skin? Researchers admit that the exact mechanism is unknown, but they do have a theory, mentioned in one of the studies. After polysaccharides are absorbed, they are taken up by the skin. There, they may stimulate fibroblast activity and help regulate cellular growth in the stratum basale, the deepest layer of the epidermis, where dividing cells are transformed into skin cells (keratinocytes).

The oral supplement costs $49.95 for 60 tablets. The manufacturer's recommended dosage is two tablets daily. Vivida 24-Hour Cream costs approximately $39.95. In addition to these products, there is a lotion, Vivida Body Lotion, priced at $29.95. Vivida products can be ordered by accessing the Web site www.theauroragrp.com.

Do not take Vivida if you have any kind of fish or shellfish allergy. If you are pregnant or lactating, talk to your physician about whether you should take an oral supplement such as Vivida.

IMEDEEN

A product similar to Vivida is Imedeen, an oral supplement made from proteins and polysaccharides extracted from fish. It also contains vitamin C, essential for the formation of collagen, and the mineral zinc, which is also involved in the synthesis of collagen.

Developed by two Swedish scientists in the early 1980s, Imedeen has also proven to be effective in treating and repairing aging skin. In a small pilot study reported in 1991, 10 women (aged 39 to 61 years old) supplemented with 500 milligrams of Imedeen for three months. By the end of the experimental period, all signs of skin damage—wrinkles, blotches, and dry skin—had greatly improved. Both skin thickness and elasticity had increased, too.

Tests continued over several years—all with similar findings: Imedeen appears to be a safe and effective treatment for photoaged skin. The only side effect that has been reported in clinical studies is a temporary skin reaction such as pimples. But these usually disappear with continued use of the supplement.

Researchers believe that Imedeen may stimulate the activity of fibroblasts; restore glycosaminoglycans, which are key structures in the skin for retaining moisture and suppleness; repair damaged collagen and elastin; and increase blood flow to skin tissue.

Marketed in more than 40 countries, Imedeen costs between $65 and $85 for a bottle of 60 tablets. The suggested dosage is two tablets a day with a glass of water. Because it is derived from fish, people with a seafood allergy should avoid Imedeen. If you are pregnant or lactating, talk to your physician about whether you should take an oral supplement such as Imedeen.

SQUALANE

The marine-based squalane oil is a desirable additive in cosmetics. As noted above, it is produced from a highly valued marine extract called squalene, which makes up 12 to 14 percent of sebum, the skin's natural lubricant. Squalane is more stable than squalene, meaning that it will not break down when exposed to air.

Scientists have found that when squalane is applied to the skin, it helps restore lost oils, thereby making the skin feel and look more supple. One reason that it is added to so many cosmetics, as well as to medical ointments, is that it increases the penetration of active ingredients into the skin. Squalane is also very gentle on the skin.

There may be antiaging properties associated with squalane, too, although these have not yet been verified scientifically. Cosmetics companies who add it to their formulations say that it preserves the skin's elasticity and helps prevent the signs of accelerated aging.

Some physicians recommend the use of squalane following chemical peels and to help moisturize the skin when using retinoids or hydroxy acids.

COSMETICS FROM THE DEAD SEA

For centuries, people have bathed in the Dead Sea to cure themselves of all sorts of diseases. Today, there are spas bordering the sea that cater to individuals seeking treatment for skin diseases such as acne as well as psoriasis, a genetic disease in which the life cycle of skin cells fast-forwards abnormally, resulting in skin eruptions and scaling. The waters of the Dead Sea are also thought to be therapeutic for allergies, arthritis, and respiratory diseases.

A landlocked salt lake between Israel and Jordan, the Dead Sea is the lowest body of water on earth. Its waters are extremely saline, with the concentration of salt increasing as the sea becomes deeper. Except for bacteria, no animal or plant life can survive in the salinity of the Dead Sea. Bathers can float easily in the sea because its high salt content buoys them up.

Legend has it that when the sea was changed into a salt lake during biblical days, creatures no longer able to thrive in the salt-laden water left behind a hormonelike substance with rejuvenating powers. That substance has not been verified by scientific research, however. Even so, the Dead Sea's minerals have been used for cosmetic purposes since ancient times. In the first century B.C., a huge beauty industry, built by Cleopatra, flourished along its shores, and according to archaeologists, the remnants of ancient cosmetic factories can still be seen. Today, more than 50 different brands of cosmetics formulated with Dead Sea minerals are sold throughout the world.

Compared with the world's major oceans and the Mediterranean Sea, the Dead Sea is infinitely richer in life-giving minerals, namely sodium, magnesium, calcium, potassium, and chloride. The water also contains salts of lithium and strontium, both thought to be beneficial to the skin.

Many Israeli researchers believe that the minerals found in the Dead Sea draw and retain moisture in the skin, as well as activate skin enzymes that help regenerate collagen and elastin. A group of Israeli scientists, writing in the *Israel Journal of Medical Sciences,* noted "that the minerals present in the water of the Dead Sea have the capability of improving skin is undeniable."

Consumers and retailers seem to agree. People who have bathed in the Dead Sea say it leaves their skin "baby-smooth." In a poll conducted by Dead Sea Laboratories, Ltd., the creator of Ahava, a top-selling Dead Sea cosmetics line, 70 percent of tourists to Israel had a positive perception of sea-mineral-based products. Eighty-six percent of the respondents stated that the cosmetics had a healthy influence on the skin.

In another survey, Israeli retailers were asked to list the benefits of products based on natural ingredients from the Dead Sea. They noted that these products contain active ingredients, engender an enthusiastic response from customers, are recommended by doctors, and have healing capabilities for healthier skin.

At least one Dead Sea product—Ahava's Mineral Skin Osmoter—has been scientifically assessed to verify its antiwrinkle benefits. Mineral Skin Osmoter is a special water containing a high concentration of Dead Sea minerals and is used as an ingredient in a variety of Ahava's skin-care products.

In this study, a well-known European dermatologic research institute, Dermatest, was asked to compare three cosmetic preparations: a placebo gel containing no active ingredients; an antiwrinkle gel, formulated with locust bean gum, glycoproteins, and fruit extracts (believed to be active antiwrinkle agents); and the same antiwrinkle gel enriched with 1 percent Osmoter.

Twenty women volunteers (aged 20 to 65) used one of these formulas daily for a month. At the end of the experimental period, Dermatest researchers measured wrinkle depth. On average, the placebo gel reduced wrinkle depth by 11 percent; the antiwrinkle gel by 27 percent; and the Osmoter-enriched gel by 40 percent. In addition to remarkably reducing wrinkles, the Dead Sea mineral formulation smoothed the skin considerably.

Dead Sea cosmetics come in various forms. There are products that contain Dead Sea mud, designed to be applied as body or face masks. These contain high concentrations of Dead Sea minerals. Other Dead Sea cosmetics are lotions, creams, or water-based solutions formulated with lower concentrations of the legendary minerals.

Numerous companies manufacture and market Dead Sea cosmetics. Among them: Ahava, Oris Cosmetics, Giora Shavit, and Neca Chemicals. In 1995, cosmetic giant L'Oréal purchased part interest in an Israeli company, Interbeauty International Cosmetics, which manufactures a line of cosmetics based on minerals and mud from the Dead Sea. The company claims that its cosmetics can improve skin elasticity, increase moisture, and restore smoothness. In general, Dead Sea cosmetics are available in major department stores, specialty boutiques, or through Web sites.

CRÈME DE LA MER

Its invention reads like a good sci-fi thriller: A NASA scientist who suffered severe burns in an accident spends 12 years and performs 6,000 experiments developing an extraordinary cream that makes skin look smoother, tighter, and remarkably younger.

The scientist was Max Huber (who died in 1991), and the cream is Crème de la Mer, which contains a seaweed fermentation made from a special seaweed harvested off the California coast only two times a year—when the material is most plentiful in nutrients. The fermentation process itself takes three to four months.

Other ingredients in Crème de la Mer include calcium, magnesium, potassium, iron, lecithin, vitamins C, D, E, and B$_{12}$, along with extracts of citrus, eucalyptus, wheat germ, alfalfa, and sunflower. Physicians have long used the cream to minimize postoperative scarring.

For many years, the product was made by Max Huber Labs. In 1995, cosmetics giant Estée Lauder bought the firm and since then has introduced a line of compatible products. This line includes the Moisturizing Lotion for normal-to-dry skin; the Oil Absorbing Lotion for normal-to-oily skins; the Cleansing Lotion and the Cleansing Gel, which prepare the skin for other Crème de la Mer treatments; the Face Serum, for delivering nutrients to the skin; the Body Serum, designed to improve overall skin condition; and the Eye Balm, created to diminish the appearance of fine lines and dark, under-the-eye discolorations.

It is the original face cream—Crème de la Mer—however, that has the most loyal following. Technically, the cream is a moisturizer, but anecdotal reports from consumers hint that it most assuredly reduces fine lines on the face. Although it can be pricey ($155 for two ounces), you don't have to use very much of it. Just a dime-sized dab will do the trick.

When to Apply Marine Cosmetics

Generally, topical marine cosmetics are formulated as moisturizers. That means you can apply them morning or evening, depending on the dryness of your skin. If you apply Renova or Retin-A at night, consider using a marine cosmetic as a daytime moisture restorer. Apply it after hydroxy acids or topical antioxidants, but before applying sunscreen.

If your skin is oily or acne-prone, try a nonoily moisturizer formulated with a marine algae extract called *phlorogine*. It is found in a product called Skin Pure from Lancaster and helps naturally regulate oiliness.

The softening action of most marine cosmetics also makes them an excellent base for makeup. If in doubt on when to apply these cosmetics, refer to the manufacturer's recommendations.

PART FIVE

Professional Procedures

PART SEVEN

Polygraph Procedures

10
Skin-Deep Beauty:
Chemical Peels

AMONG the best ways to banish deep-set wrinkles and rejuvenate your skin is a procedure known as a *chemical peel.* It involves the application of a liquid solution containing alpha hydroxy acids, trichloroacetic acid (TCA), or phenol to remove the top layers of skin. In effect, the solution produces inflammation similar to a sunburn, and, accordingly, the top layers of your skin peel off.

As part of the natural healing process, the peeled skin is eventually swapped with a new, smoother layer of skin. Depending on the strength of the solution, collagen in the dermis is regenerated, too, making your skin appear tighter and more youthful.

Chemical peels are categorized as "light" (or "superficial"), "medium," or "deep." These designations refer to the depth at which the peeling liquid sinks into the skin. Different types of liquid penetrate the skin at different levels. Alpha hydroxy peels, for example, are the mildest, peeling off only the topmost layers of skin. At the other end of the spectrum is the phenol peel, which penetrates quite deeply and can achieve rather dramatic results in rejuvenating the skin. The cost of a chemical peel varies considerably, but ranges from $760 to $1,270, according to the American Society of Plastic Surgeons.

Both widely available and popular, chemical peels have been around for centuries. Ancient Egyptian writings dating back about 3,500 years ago record instructions for applying peeling chemicals to the skin. In the early 1900s, chemical peels were widely used in Europe, particularly for removing acne scars. They were first introduced to the United States with the influx of German dermatologists in the 1920s and 1930s. The procedure virtually disappeared from the scene in the 1940s and 1950s as a result of complications caused by nonmedical peelers and the social pressures of intervening wars. But with the development of improved TCA and phenol peels in the 1960s and alpha hydroxy peels in the 1980s, the procedure regained its former popularity and today is a highly regarded treatment for wrinkles and aging skin.

The various types of chemical peels are discussed below, along with guidelines for deciding if a peel is right for your skin.

ALPHA HYDROXY (AHA) PEELS

With AHA peels, solutions of glycolic acid, lactic acid, or other fruit acids are applied to your skin to slough off the outer two or three layers of the topmost epidermis (the stratum corneum). These peels are appropriate if you have mild sun damage. They can work in concert with a skin-care regimen that includes tretinoin and sunscreens.

Ultimately, the procedure minimizes fine lines, smoothes out dry, rough skin, reduces pore size, and corrects the texture of sun-damaged skin. AHA peels are also used to treat acne. When mixed with a bleaching agent, these peels help improve age spots and erase blotchiness.

AHA peels are often used by plastic surgeons and dermatologists as a pretreatment for other cosmetic procedures
such as deeper peels or for laser resurfacing.

The improved outer appearance of the skin is due to the
effects of AHA on the deeper layers of the skin. Scientific
experiments have revealed that AHA peels increase the
thickness of collagen in the dermis, plus reverse the age-
related thinning of the epidermis and dermis.

The most common peeling agent is glycolic acid, usually in concentrations ranging from 40 to 70 percent. Another agent is Jessner's solution, formulated with 14
percent lactic acid, 14 percent resorcinol (a phenollike
acid), and 14 percent salicylic acid, a beta hydroxy acid. In
research, salicylic acid has been shown to work slightly
better than glycolic acid. Salicylic acid sloughs off more
outer skin cells and produces smoother skin.

AHA peels are available in salons, administered by
trained estheticians, or in clinics, performed by plastic surgeons or dermatologists. Generally, physicians employ 50
to 70 percent concentrations, usually composed of glycolic
acid, although other peeling agents may be used. The pH
of these solutions ranges from 0.08 to 2.75. For trained estheticians in salons, the FDA allows a concentration of glycolic acid or lactic acid of up to 30 percent and a pH of 3.0
or higher. An AHA peel should always be performed by a
trained professional.

Prior to Your AHA Peel

Quite probably, your physician or skin-care professional
will first obtain a complete history to determine whether
you have any conditions that make it ill advised to undergo
an AHA peel. An AHA peel should not be performed if
you:

◊ Have active cold sores (herpes simplex) on your face.

◊ Suffer from facial warts.

◊ Are pregnant or lactating.

◊ Take the oral retinoid Accutane. (It increases the risk of scarring.)

◊ Have a history of sun allergies.

◊ Have a sunburn.

◊ Have experienced a bad reaction to a prior facial peel.

◊ Have recently had any type of facial surgery.

In addition, you may be asked about any medications you're taking. Aspirin, warfarin (Coumadin), and photosensitizing agents, such as tetracycline, may affect the peel and your recovery time. Thus, it's wise to avoid these products for a few weeks prior to your peel.

You may be given an AHA lotion to apply once or twice daily at home for a few weeks. It helps thin out the topmost layer of the epidermis and gets your skin accustomed to the peeling solution. One week prior to the peel, you may be asked to stop using various products, including hair dyes, permanent-wave or hair-straightening treatments, facial masks, waxing, or loofah sponges.

During the AHA Peel

Arrive for your peel without makeup, lotions, cologne, sunscreen, or contact lenses. Your face should be fully cleansed.

To remove dead skin cells, excess oil, and residual makeup, the physician or esthetician will wash your face with a special cleanser, such as an enzyme solution. Next, your skin may be "dermaplaned" with a special scalpel to remove any dead skin cells.

The peeling agent is applied to your face with a cotton applicator, fine brush, or by gloved hand. As the solution is placed on your face, you may experience some stinging. Often, an electric fan will be directed toward your face to divert vapors and help alleviate stinging.

The procedure is virtually painless, however, and no anesthetic is required. The solution is left on your face for up to seven minutes. Afterward your face is coated with a solution of sodium bicarbonate or other agent to neutralize the peel. Next, your face will be rinsed, and cold compresses may be applied. The esthetician will then apply a moisturizing sunscreen to your face.

After Your AHA Peel

After-care for an AHA peel is critical. Because peels make your skin more susceptible to sunlight, you'll be instructed to wear sunscreen with an SPF of 15 or higher. You may have to use some type of lubricating lotion to enhance the healing process. Applying petroleum jelly to affected areas minimizes crusting and helps the skin peel more evenly. Following your peel, it may be a day or two before you can start wearing makeup again, but generally, you can go about your normal routine.

Some skin specialists recommend the use of an AHA-based facial wash or cream once or twice a day to keep skin smooth—a practice shown in research to further minimize fine lines. Use a 10 percent AHA product for best results. If you're under the care of a dermatologist or plastic surgeon, Renova or a bleaching agent may be prescribed to supplement your antiwrinkle regimen.

The positive effects of an AHA peel do not last. You'll need to have a series of peels on a periodic basis to maintain your smoother-looking skin. Several treatments—usually weekly or bimonthly—are required to achieve the desired cosmetic results.

SAFETY AND SIDE EFFECTS

AHA peels have virtually no side effects, with the possible exception of redness, flakiness, and mild crusting. A study conducted at the University of California School of Medicine found that stronger AHA solutions (70 percent with a pH below 2) produced more tissue damage and caused crusting of the skin. The researchers pointed out that the use of lower-concentration solutions (50 percent) with a pH above 2 is safer and more advisable.

If you are susceptible to cold sores, however, peels can cause flare-ups. These can be prevented by taking a prescription antiviral drug called Acyclovir. Discuss this option with your physician.

TRICHLOROACETIC ACID (TCA) PEELS

TCA is a derivative of acetic acid, the chief acid found in vinegar. Used in concentrations between 35 and 50 percent, TCA produces a medium-depth peel on the face. The higher the concentration, the deeper the peel. In smaller concentrations (10 to 25 percent), it can be applied to the neck, where undesirable signs of aging can be quite noticeable. Increasingly, TCA peels are being used to rejuvenate the skin of the eyelids, which turns papery and droopy with age.

Normally, a liquid TCA solution is applied to the face during a peel. A newer form of application is the TCA Masque, a cream formulation available in 11 percent and 16.9 percent concentrations. Applied by a physician or specially trained nurse, it is a claylike mask that dries on the skin and remains there for three to five minutes. A study conducted at the University of South Florida in Tampa found that the TCA Masque eliminated fine wrinkles and freshened the skin. Some physicians use a combination of glycolic acid and TCA in their peeling solutions and masks.

TCA peels are performed in a physician's office. No anesthetic is required.

You may want to consider a TCA peel if you desire to:

◊ Smooth out larger wrinkles.

◊ Remove superficial blemishes.

◊ Correct blotchiness or other pigmentation problems.

Like AHA peels, TCA peels thicken and rejuvenate the skin by regenerating collagen. The effect of peels on elastin—the structural protein that gives your skin its youthful bounce—has not been well studied, though. In fact, research conducted on Yucatán mini-pigs at the Stanford University Medical School in Palo Alto, California, demonstrated that applications of TCA had no effect on the structure, arrangement, or quality of elastin fibers in skin. (The skin of mini-pigs is similar to human skin, which is why these animals were used in the experiment.)

Prior to Your TCA Peel

As with an AHA peel, your physician will take your medical history. A TCA peel should not be performed if you:

◊ Have active cold sores on your face.

◊ Suffer from facial warts.

◊ Are pregnant or lactating.

◊ Take the oral retinoid Accutane.

◊ Have a history of sun allergies.

◊ Have a sunburn.

◊ Have experienced a bad reaction to a prior facial peel.

◊ Have recently had any type of facial surgery.

Your physician may prescribe Renova or Retin-A to be used for four to six weeks prior to the TCA peel. This medication helps prepare your skin for the procedure.

During Your TCA Peel

Although application procedures may differ from physician to physician, here's generally what to expect during a TCA peel: Prior to the peel, your physician will wash your face to remove any dirt and oil. Next, a light AHA solution is applied to exfoliate the skin and help increase the penetration of the TCA peel.

The TCA solution is then painted on your skin. It will burn a bit and frost over, making your skin feel tight. Two or three coats of TCA may be required. Your physician may then place cold compresses on your face, followed by an application of Polysporin, an over-the-counter antibiotic. The procedure lasts 10 to 15 minutes.

After Your TCA Peel

Following your peel, you may feel some discomfort, which can generally be eased with aspirin or other over-the-counter pain relievers. Initially, your face may be slightly red, then turn a tannish color. The tan discoloration may last two or three days. Next, you'll notice that your face will start peeling—a process that lasts five days, on average. You can resume wearing makeup in approximately one week. Newer, fresher-looking skin will be evident in a week to 10 days.

You will be instructed to keep your face clean with regular washing and to liberally apply a moisturizing lotion to lubricate the skin. Research indicates that the use of a moisturizer following a TCA peel accelerates healing. Your physician will recommend an appropriate product. In addition, you must wear a high-SPF sunscreen every day for several months.

SAFETY AND SIDE EFFECTS

TCA is not absorbed into your system; it works only at skin level and therefore does not produce any toxic side effects. Like an AHA peel, a TCA peel may cause cold sores to erupt.

The results of a TCA peel are more enduring than those of an AHA peel, but they are not permanent. Two or more TCA peels may be required, but should be spaced out over several months. A series of TCA peels should be performed only every couple of years.

PHENOL PEELS

Deep peels use phenol (carbolic acid) in varying concentrations. The most commonly used phenol peel is known as the Baker formula, which contains a concentration of 45 to 50 percent phenol. Also used in the formula is croton oil, an irritant that induces blistering to allow better penetration of the phenol into the dermis; Septisol, a liquid soap that prevents overpenetration of phenol and neutralizes the irritant effects of the formula; and distilled water.

Cosmetically, a phenol peel is a good option if you want

to minimize deeper, coarser wrinkles without resorting to a face-lift or other cosmetic surgical procedure. Your complexion must be fair and on the dry side, too. Phenol peels lighten the skin considerably. Thus, if your skin is light already, there will be less contrast following treatment. Dark-skinned women are not good candidates for phenol peels. Also, dry skin absorbs the phenol solution better than oily skin.

Most phenol peels are performed on the entire face. However, the solution can be applied to smaller portions of the face, such as the upper lip. Usually, only one peel is needed to obtain the desired cosmetic improvement.

Prior to Your Phenol Peel

Your physician will obtain a complete family and medical history, with special attention to allergies and heart or kidney problems. (Phenol is potentially toxic and can aggravate certain medical problems.)

In addition to taking a history, your physician may obtain a baseline electrocardiogram, a complete blood count, and other routine laboratory tests. Your physician will probably photograph your face, too. During this visit, you should get answers to all questions about the procedure and sign a consent form.

If no problems arise, a small amount of the phenol solution will be applied to an inconspicuous spot, such as the hairline of your upper forehead, and observed for several weeks to note any adverse reactions.

If the procedure is a thumbs-up, your physician may recommend the use of Renova or Retin-A, applied nightly, for several weeks prior to your peel. This medication promotes the shedding of dead skin cells (corneocytes) on the outer layer of the epidermis, which leads to better absorption of the solution during the peel.

In all likelihood, your physician will tell you to avoid

aspirin and other medications that affect normal blood clotting. If you smoke, you'll be advised to quit about a week or two before the peel, because smoking restricts blood circulation in the skin and interferes with healing.

During Your Phenol Peel

A phenol peel is performed as an outpatient procedure, but in an operating room. You'll lie on a table with your head slightly elevated. You may be given a sedative and a pain reliever. A local anesthetic is sometimes used to relieve discomfort.

Your face will be cleansed with either soap and water, or with a solvent such as alcohol or acetone. Use of solvents helps achieve a more even distribution of phenol across your face during the peel.

Peeling is done in sections. Using a cotton-tipped applicator, your physician will uniformly apply the solution to each section of your face, usually beginning with your forehead and progressing to the upper temples, the cheeks, and so forth.

After one section is coated, the physician waits about 15 minutes before coating another one. This technique helps prevent adverse reactions. During application, the physician takes care to ensure that the solution evenly coats the depth of each wrinkle. As the phenol contacts the skin, your skin will turn a frosty white. You'll experience a burning sensation that lasts up to 30 seconds. The entire peel takes 90 minutes to two hours, on average.

After Your Phenol Peel

You'll be observed for 30 minutes following the procedure. (Some patients may be required to stay overnight for a day or two for observation.)

Following the 30-minute observation period, your

physician will apply a dressing to your face. It consists of layers of a special tape that should stay in place for 24 to 48 hours. Someone should drive you home afterward because your eyes may be swollen shut, and you may be in pain.

At home, you should rest in bed in a semireclining or sitting position and take mild pain relievers to ease any discomfort. To minimize facial movement, your physician will advise a liquid diet, consumed with a straw, and recommend that you limit your talking. Be sure to follow to the letter all your physician's postoperative instructions.

After about 24 hours, your skin will start to exude a thin, watery liquid as part of the healing process. This will loosen the tape. You can gently remove it while showering, or if you prefer, have it taken off in your physician's office. Your skin will be quite red, swollen, and irritated, resembling a second-degree burn.

Depending on your physician's instructions, you'll be advised to cleanse your face frequently with cool tap water, followed by the application of a nonalcohol lubricant or an antibiotic ointment. A mild cortisone ointment might be prescribed as well, to minimize inflammation. Scab formation is normal. Do not pick any scabs, however, or you could leave scars on your face. After 10 to 12 days, you should begin using a physician-recommended moisturizer and sunscreen.

Avoid alcohol for several weeks, since drinking alcoholic beverages may prolong or worsen facial redness.

The healing process following a phenol peel is quite lengthy. In roughly two to three weeks, you can resume your normal routine. It takes nearly three months for skin redness to disappear. You can camouflage the redness by using a green-based, hypoallergenic makeup.

Unlike light and medium peels, the results of a phenol peel are more permanent—and quite dramatic. Your new skin will appear younger, more glowing, and very smooth.

Over time, however, new wrinkles will appear as part of the normal aging process.

SAFETY AND SIDE EFFECTS

With a phenol peel, there is the risk of infection, scarring, and abnormal or uneven skin-color changes. Cold sores may flare up, too. Although rare, heart irregularities may develop during the procedure.

A phenol peel permanently lightens your skin, and your face will never tan because it loses its ability to make pigment. If you have a phenol peel, you must always wear sunscreen because your skin is now highly sensitive to the sun.

FINDING A SPECIALIST

If you wish to have a chemical peel, consult a physician or esthetician who is qualified, trained, and experienced in these techniques. Superficial peels, such as AHA peels, are generally performed by estheticians. The medium- and deeper-depth peels should be performed by a board-certified dermatologist or plastic surgeon.

11

Wrinkle Fillers

D O you long for the days when your face was virtually creaseless, plumped up, and youthful?

That was before aging, gravity, sunlight, and years of facial movement began to break down your skin's underlying structures—including collagen, elastin, and fat. Now deeper wrinkles, sagging skin, and sunken areas of the face have replaced the supple smoothness of youth.

Among the ways to fill in those lines and plump up facial caverns is through the use of injectable fillers, a cosmetic-surgery procedure that has been growing in popularity but is not new. The practice of injecting fillers into the body has been with us for more than 100 years. In the early part of the twentieth century, physicians injected patients with mineral oil, paraffin, and other oils and waxes to correct facial deformities, enlarge breasts, and perform other corrective procedures. But these early, primitive operations were fraught with complications. Fortunately, though, the cosmetic use of injectables has come a long way since then.

Today, plastic surgeons and dermatologists have a whole lineup of viable substances they can inject under your skin to help you regain the look of youth. These filler substances prop up depressed wrinkles, push them outward, and thus make wrinkles less noticeable. Some fillers are designed to mimic the properties of collagen and elastin in the dermis— that is, provide strength and resilience. Wrinkle fillers are used alone, or often in combination with other procedures, such as skin resurfacing or a face-lift. The following are fillers used in cosmetic surgery:

BOVINE COLLAGEN

Collagen is the naturally occurring structural protein found in the skin, joints, ligaments, and bones. It is the most common protein in the body.

The most widely used injectable form is derived from bovine (cow) collagen in a purification process that produces a collagen similar to that found in our own bodies. In the United States, three forms of bovine collagen—Zyderm I, Zyderm II, and Zyplast—are officially authorized by the FDA as devices (not drugs) for implantation in the human body. Approved since 1981, they are used to fill in deep wrinkles and scars on the face, neck, back, and chest.

Another cosmetic use of injected bovine collagen is to enhance the lips by giving them a voluptuous, pouty look made popular by models and actresses. This use, however, is not approved by the FDA.

Injected bovine collagen is believed to work not only by initially plumping up the skin underneath but also by stimulating the creation of new collagen in the dermis—a response that has been verified in research studies.

To date, well more than a half million people have been treated with bovine collagen. There are nearly 55,000 procedures performed annually, according to the American Society of Plastic Surgeons.

For this procedure, you will pay between $600 and $1,300

for treatment of the upper lips; between $900 and $1,700 for the forehead; and between $800 and $1,500 for crow's-feet.

Prior to the Procedure

Your cosmetic surgeon will take a complete medical history to rule out any allergies or medical conditions that could cause trouble. This procedure is not recommended for anyone who has a history of autoimmune diseases, connective-tissue disease, allergies to beef or bovine products, or sensitivity to lidocaine (the anesthetic used in the procedure). If pregnant, you should not undergo this procedure.

Before the treatment, you'll be tested for a possible allergic reaction to bovine collagen, the chief complication of the procedure. About 3 percent of the population is allergic to collagen.

One month prior to the procedure, your cosmetic surgeon will perform an allergy skin test by injecting a small amount of collagen in your forearm and watching for a reaction. Usually, any response will show up in 48 hours, although in some patients, the reaction appears three weeks later. Signs of an allergic reaction include redness, rash, hives, itching, swelling, joint or muscle pain, or other untoward symptoms. These symptoms can usually be resolved by taking oral antihistamines and topical or oral steroids. Your physician will determine the best treatment for your case.

During Treatment

Injectable procedures are usually performed in the cosmetic surgeon's office-based facility. The anesthetic lidocaine is combined with the collagen to help numb any pain. The solution also contains some salt water.

For patients who are very sensitive to pain, a topical anesthetic might be used along with a sedative. Your surgeon will determine the best course of action for your individual situation.

During the procedure, the surgeon inserts a fine needle into your skin at selected treatment sites and injects the collagen. Full-face treatment may require numerous needle sticks. You may feel some minor stinging or burning. After the injections, the surgeon may massage the surface of the skin.

After the Treatment

You may feel some minor discomfort, including stinging or throbbing at the treated sites. Some patients have swelling, bruising, or redness, but these symptoms are rare and usually disappear within 24 hours. Any scabs that form over the needle-insertion points should heal rapidly.

Your surgeon may advise that you avoid all facial movements (including speaking) for four hours following treatment. Stay out of the sun for at least two days after treatment. You can resume wearing makeup within a couple of days.

Generally, there are few risks and complications with this procedure, particularly if it is performed by an experienced, board-certified surgeon. If you have any symptoms that do not resolve, however, contact your surgeon.

Some cosmetic surgeons may recommend that you have repeated injections two to four weeks apart to achieve the desired cosmetic effect. The cosmetic benefits of this treatment, however, do not last because the body breaks down and assimilates bovine collagen. Zyderm I and Zyderm II, according to medical studies, will last up to three months, while Zyplast lasts longer. Thus, you may have to undergo touch-ups every three to twelve months, depending upon the recommendations of your surgeon, your response to treatment, and your desire to maintain the cosmetic benefits.

FAT TRANSPLANTATION

Since the nineteenth century, fat transplants have been used to plump up soft tissue in various parts of the body. In the modern-day version of this procedure, fat cells are extracted from your abdomen, thighs, or buttocks, then reinjected beneath the skin on your face so that they can settle into the dermis. The extracted fat helps fill in sunken cheeks, plump up marionette lines between the nose and mouth, decrease frown lines on the forehead, and augment the lips.

The procedure costs roughly $750 when a few sites are treated; $4,000 for a full-face treatment.

Prior to the Procedure

As with any cosmetic procedure, your surgeon will take your medical history and evaluate whether the procedure is appropriate for your case. If you have a bleeding disorder or diabetes, fat transplantation may be off-limits. Unlike bovine collagen, allergic reactions are usually not a problem with injected fat, because it is taken from your own body.

During Treatment

The first step is the removal of fat from another region of your body—known as the "donor" site. The donor site is numbed with local anesthetic. The surgeon inserts either a syringe or a narrow tube called a *cannula* into the locally anesthetized area. The cannula suctions out fat cells. The extracted fat is then processed into an injectable form and injected into *recipient sites* on the face, which have also been numbed with local anesthetic. The surgeon will probably overfill areas to allow for proper fat absorption and contouring.

After the Treatment

Your face may be a bit puffy as a result of the overfilling, but this condition will subside in two to three days, on average. Normally, you can get back to your regular routine right away. Recovery time may be longer if a larger portion of your face was treated. You may also have visible puncture holes on your face at the injection sites, and these may persist for several days, or even a few weeks. It is a good idea to avoid sun exposure for two days and apply sunscreen liberally thereafter.

Be sure to follow your surgeon's instructions to the letter and report any unusual or lingering side effects.

As with collagen injections, the results of fat transplantation do not last indefinitely but taper off in three months to a year, depending on how fast the fat is absorbed by your body. You will need additional treatments to maintain the benefits.

OTHER FILLER MATERIALS

While bovine collagen and human fat are the most widely used, other injectable filler substances are being employed to rejuvenate the face. Here's a rundown:

Fibril

Fibril is a gelatin powder reconstituted with your own blood and injected into wrinkle or scar-bearing sites. It was developed in the 1980s as an alternative to bovine collagen, primarily as a filler substance for scars. The gelatin powder is derived from the collagen of pigs.

Fibril also contains a substance called *epsilon aminocaproic acid,* which together with the gelatin powder and blood mimics the normal process of blood clotting and wound healing. The net effect is to stimulate the formation of new collagen in the treated skin.

Most of the research with Fibril has focused on its ability to correct depressed scars. Other research has targeted wrinkle treatment. In one study, researchers found that in 100 patients treated with Fibril, 25 to 35 percent maintained smoother skin for an entire year.

There are very few known side effects associated with Fibril. Even so, some skin researchers feel that Fibril treatment causes greater swelling and redness than bovine collagen injections do. Compared with other filler procedures, larger needles are required to place the material in the dermis. Thus, you may experience more pain and discomfort.

On a positive note: Some patients who are allergic to bovine collagen may not allergic to pig collagen, making Fibril an option if you're sensitive to Zyderm or Zyplast. What's more, injected Fibril reportedly lasts slightly longer than injected collagen.

The average cost of treatment is approximately $735, according to the American Society of Plastic Surgeons. If you're thinking about having Fibril injections, discuss the risks and benefits with a qualified cosmetic surgeon.

Human Collagen Fillers

Cosmetic surgeons have long considered implanting human collagen to be the ideal way to treat damaged skin. There's less chance of degradation in the body, allergic reactions, or rejection of the implanted material. Thus newer procedures have evolved, using the patient's own collagen or collagen from skin tissue that would normally have been discarded from other cosmetic procedures. Skin is sent to a special lab, and its collagen is extracted and processed. The lab stores the collagen for future use and later returns it to the surgeon in preloaded syringes.

One of these procedures uses a human collagen called

Autologen. This filler is harvested from your own skin, prepared at a special lab to extract your natural collagen, processed into a liquid form, and then injected into the desired area at a later date.

Autologen is employed to correct deep facial lines. The cost of the procedure is approximately $800 to $1,000 per session.

Prior to the procedure, a local anesthetic is applied to the injection site. Using a small needle, the cosmetic surgeon injects the collagen into the dermis. Results are visible immediately. Clinical research shows that a series of three Autologen treatments can keep the skin virtually wrinkle-free for more than one year.

Although you may experience some temporary swelling and minor bruising after the procedure, you can resume your normal activities within a few hours, on average. Your processed collagen can be stored for up to five years, in case you wish to repeat the procedure.

A similar filler is Isolagen, made from cloned collagen-producing cells extracted from your own skin. To initiate this procedure, your surgeon will remove a tiny piece of your skin and send it to the Isolagen lab for processing. After a few weeks the lab returns your Isolagen, which contains live cells, to your surgeon. A series of three injections is required, and your skin will continue to improve after the last injection as the cloned cells manufacture new collagen. You may need additional treatments in the future to maintain the cosmetic benefit. Isolagen costs $1,000 to $1,500 per session.

Dermalogen, another human collagen, is made from human cadaver skin donated to tissue banks and prepared using a patented process that sterilizes the skin tissue. Injected into the skin, Dermalogen is used to treat smile lines, wrinkles around the upper lip, frown lines, marionette lines, and depressed scars. The cost is approximately $750 to $1,100 per session.

Typically, you'll require two to three treatments over a

three-month period. Studies show that the positive effects of a Dermalogen injection may last for up to two years.

AlloDerm Grafts

Available since 1994, AlloDerm is derived from human cadaver skin that has been specially sterilized and processed to remove all cells while preserving only a collagen matrix, termed a *graft*. This matrix provides a scaffolding upon which new skin cells can grow.

After numbing the skin with local anesthesia, the cosmetic surgeon makes tiny incisions on either side of the wrinkle or scar and implants the graft under the skin between the incisions. The incisions are sutured shut with a transparent material that is removed several days later. Eventually, the graft becomes a part of your own tissue. Cosmetically, the graft smoothes out deep lines. It has also been used successfully in lip-augmentation procedures.

Because it is human tissue, AlloDerm does not normally provoke allergic reactions. Usually, you don't have to have skin test prior to the operation. And unlike injected fat or collagen, the graft does not degrade with time. Thus there is usually no need for additional treatments.

The average cost of an AlloDerm graft is $1,000.

Gore-Tex

Gore-Tex is a synthetic material that has been used for more than thirty years on patients undergoing cardiovascular and abdominal surgery as well as kidney transplants. More recently, it has been employed in cosmetic surgery for nasal and facial reconstruction and for the treatment of wrinkles because it is a pliable material that blends well with your own tissue. Gore-Tex is used primarily to enhance areas around the lip, but can prop up areas such as the chin that tend to sag and recede with age.

Gore-Tex implantation is performed as an outpatient procedure. Prior to the procedure, your skin is numbed with a topical anesthetic, and lidocaine (another anesthetic) is injected into the site to provide additional anesthesia.

The surgeon passes the Gore-Tex implant through a needle and threads it underneath the skin to fill in deep wrinkles. The entrance and exit incisions are sutured shut or sealed with a laser.

Following the procedure, you may experience some swelling, which can be eased by cold compresses. Your surgeon may also prescribe antibiotics to prevent the possibility of infection.

Side effects are rare, although there is the risk of infection and the slight chance that your body will reject the implant. If rejection occurs, the threads will be taken out. There may also be some slight asymmetry.

The results of Gore-Tex are permanent because the material does not dissolve, nor is it reabsorbed by the body. The beauty of Gore-Tex is that it stimulates the body to form new collagen around the implant for additional smoothness.

The average cost for a Gortex implant is $2,500 for one lip, $4,000 for both.

Hylaform Gel

This filler is made from a naturally occurring lubricant called *hyaluronic acid* found in skin and other tissues, but gradually lost with age. Hylaform gel uses hyaluronic acid obtained from animals. Cosmetically, it is injected under the skin to fill in and smooth out scars and wrinkles as well as to augment the lips. Treatment with Hylaform gel is available in Europe and Canada, but not yet in the United States.

Hylaform gel has been clinically tested for its effectiveness against wrinkles and scars. In one study, 80 percent of the patients expressed moderate to high satisfaction three months after treatment. Another study found that the detectable benefits of Hylaform gel injections lasted nearly twice as long (one year) as those of injected collagen (22 weeks).

During the procedure, the surgeon will numb the skin with a local anesthetic and make a series of injections at the sites to be treated. The procedure takes approximately 30 minutes. There is little or no recovery time. Some patients, however, may experience swelling, redness, or other symptoms of irritation.

Hylaform is gradually degraded by the body, so you'll require follow-up treatments two to three times a year. Because this treatment is not yet widely available, you'll have to discuss costs with a cosmetic surgeon who performs it.

BOTOX

Not a true filler but an injectable antiwrinkle agent nonetheless, Botox is a protein that arrests muscular contractions around the injected site. When certain facial muscles stop contracting, you can't frown or squint. Consequently, the progressive formation of wrinkles is halted temporarily. This ultimately softens the appearance of fine lines and wrinkles. Generally, cosmetic surgeons feel that Botox works best on lines of expression, namely crow's-feet, frown lines, and forehead wrinkles. Nearly 500,000 treatments are performed annually, according to the American Society of Plastic Surgeons.

Botox is derived from one of the world's most potent poisons, botulinum toxin. Botox, however, has been genetically altered and does not contain any toxic bacteria.

Botox was first employed medically in the 1970s to treat strabismus, a condition in which the muscles controlling one eyeball are imbalanced and vision is compromised. Physicians then began to use Botox cosmetically in the late eighties and early nineties to correct crow's-feet and to treat the *glabella,* the wrinkle-prone area between the eyebrows. Today, the use of Botox is often combined with laser resurfacing in facial-rejuvenation procedures.

Using a very thin needle, the surgeon injects Botox at various sites on the face. Neither a local anesthetic nor a sedative is used because the needle is so small, and there is hardly any discomfort during the procedure. You may have some mild bruising, which disappears within a few days. Normally, you can return to your regular activities right away.

After the injection, the muscle underneath the injection site relaxes. Your skin will begin to smooth out over a five-day period as a result. The relaxation lasts approximately six months, so you'll need to have follow-up treatments.

There are very few side effects associated with Botox treatments. However, if it is injected too close to your upper eyelids, they may droop—a side effect that may take several months to resolve.

Do not have Botox injections if you are pregnant or suffer from a nervous-system disease, neuromuscular disease, or a known allergy to components of Botox such as saline solution or human albumin. Botox injections may not be suitable if you're an actor or TV personality who relies on facial expressiveness to perform, since the treatment temporarily paralyzes facial muscles.

For this treatment, expect to pay from $400 to $900 for crow's-feet, from $600 to $1,300 for forehead wrinkles.

FINDING A SPECIALIST

If you are considering an injectable wrinkle treatment, consult a board-certified plastic surgeon who is experienced in these procedures. An excellent resource for locating a specialist is www.plasticsurgery.org, the Web site of the American Society of Plastic Surgeons.

12

Antiaging Breakthroughs: Skin Resurfacing

I F you want to obliterate deeper wrinkles and other imperfections but think it's impossible to do without having a face-lift—think again. *Surgical resurfacing* may be an option worth considering. It has a proven track record for removing wrinkles and scars, and is far less invasive than a face-lift. In essence, this method refinishes, or scrapes away, the top layers of your skin using a surgical instrument or a special type of laser. In this chapter, we'll look at the various types of resurfacing procedures available—how they work, what to expect, and whether you're a good candidate.

DERMABRASION

Whereas a chemical peel uses a caustic solution to remove wrinkles, dermabrasion employs a special instrument. Dermabrasion, however, can remove more of the wrinkle than a chemical peel can. Some physicians prefer dermabrasion over chemical peels because the depth of tissue removal can be better controlled. With dermabrasion, there is no absorption of chemicals, namely phenol, into the body.

Prior to the Procedure

To avoid potential complications, research and locate a plastic surgeon or dermatologist who is board certified and experienced in performing dermabrasions.

Your physician will take a complete medical history, conduct a physical examination, and photograph your face. You may be given guidelines on what to eat or drink prior to the procedure, as well as what medications to avoid. Aspirin, vitamin E, and certain medications interfere with normal blood clotting, so you'll probably be asked to stop taking them a few weeks prior to having dermabrasion. If you're a smoker, you'll have to quit a week or two before the operation, because smoking interferes with healing.

Certain individuals are not good candidates for dermabrasion. Having active acne, herpes, a skin burn, or other skin problems poses special risks, since you're more vulnerable to infection and its spread. Quite probably, your physician will recommend that you postpone the procedure until your skin has healed or cleared up.

Skin type and color affect whether you're a suitable candidate because dermabrasion may permanently lighten or discolor your skin—a troublesome side effect if you have black, Asian, or otherwise dark skin. Usually, people with dark complexions are advised not to undergo dermabrasion.

If you plan to have dermabrasion, be sure to make arrangements for someone to drive you home afterward, because your face may swell and you may experience mild pain.

The average cost of a dermabrasion is $1,775, according to the American Society of Plastic Surgeons.

During the Procedure

Dermabrasion is generally performed at a physician's facility, an outpatient surgical center, or a hospital. A local anesthetic will be applied to your face to numb the area, and you may be given a sedative for relaxation. In some cases, the physician may administer a general anesthetic.

Using a special, motorized wire brush or a burr containing diamond particles, the physician will scrape away the topmost layer of your skin to make wrinkles and other facial defects less visible. Dermabrasion can take from a few minutes to an hour and a half, depending on how much skin is involved. Afterward the physician may apply a special ointment or dressing to your skin.

After the Procedure

Your skin will be very red and swollen, and you may feel some pain. Taking a mild pain reliever will ease your discomfort. The redness and swelling should subside within a week or less.

As a natural part of the healing process, expect a scab or crust to form over the treated skin. Applying a physician-recommended ointment will minimize scab formation.

Although your skin will be pinkish for several weeks, the good news is that firmer, younger-looking skin is forming underneath the scab. In about three months, your skin should be completely healed.

Be sure to follow your physician's instructions for skin care following dermabrasion. Usually, it will be about two weeks before you can return to work. You should also protect your skin from the sun for at least six months.

Should the treated area ever worsen, however, notify your physician immediately because abnormal scars may be forming.

Side Effects

Dermabrasion carries few risks when it is performed by an experienced, board-certified physician. The most common side effect is a change in skin color. Your skin may become lighter or blotchy, or it may darken, particularly if you expose it to sunlight in the weeks following the procedure.

Some people develop whiteheads after dermabrasion; these can be treated with regular cleansing. Your pores may look larger than usual because of swelling, but they will return to normal size as the healing process continues.

Your skin will begin to look younger and more revitalized in approximately three months. Taking good care of your skin with Renova or Retin-A, hydroxy acids, sunscreen, and other topical cosmetics will help preserve the benefits of dermabrasion. At some future date, you may want to repeat the procedure. Discuss this option with your physician.

MICRODERMABRASION

You may have seen something called *microdermabrasion,* advertised in the salon where you get your hair styled or your nails manicured. It goes by other names, too: microabrasion, derma peel, lunchtime peel, or power peel. Used in Europe for more than a decade, microdermabrasion is a less aggressive form of dermabrasion that has been available in the United States for just a few years. It is performed by physicians, as well as by estheticians, to remove fine lines, shrink pore size, reduce acne scars, and improve the color and texture of skin. It also helps the skin better absorb other antiaging treatments, such as tretinoin (Renova or Retin-A).

Microdermabrasion is performed in a physician's office or a skin-care salon and requires no anesthesia. With this procedure, sterile sandlike particles of aluminum oxide are blown over your skin several times, then removed with a vacuum device. This sandblastinglike technique removes the outer layers of the epidermis so they can be replaced with new, younger-looking skin. The procedure takes just 20 to 30 minutes.

According to dermatologist Mark Rubin, M.D., in a news release issued by the American Academy of Dermatology: "What we're accomplishing with microabrasion is not only removing some of the damaged skin, but stimulating new cell growth as well. Research has shown that repetitive, superficial abrasions can create significant new cell growth."

Microdermabrasion is painless. Unlike full-fledged dermabrasion, there are virtually no aftereffects, with the exception of a little redness or swelling in the skin. This can last from an hour to 24 hours. The skin does not form a crust.

There is no lengthy recovery time, either. You can return to work the next day.

For best results, however, you should undergo a series of microdermabrasion treatments—up to five sessions a week. Expect to pay between $125 and $200 for a single treatment. Microdermabrasion works best if your skin is on the fair side.

LASER RESURFACING

A skin-rejuvenation technique that is growing in popularity is laser resurfacing, also called a *laser peel;* approximately 160,000 procedures are performed each year. With this technique, a cosmetic surgeon uses a highly focused laser beam to remove areas of wrinkled or damaged skin. Laser resurfacing can be used to treat the entire face or portions of the face by zapping troublesome spots such as crow's-feet or laugh lines. It is also employed to remove acne scars. The procedure is often used in conjunction with a face-lift, eyelid surgery, or other cosmetic operations.

Laser resurfacing works in the following manner: Aimed at the skin, a very strong beam of laser energy vaporizes the water inside cells. The cells shrink, then disappear. This ultimately causes the skin to tighten. During the healing process, new collagen is formed, and elastin fibers are restored. The result is smoother, firmer, and more youthful-looking skin.

Laser resurfacing can be light, medium, or deep. With a light laser peel, the cosmetic surgeon makes fewer laser passes over the skin, and usually, only the epidermis is treated. Medium laser peels affect the epidermis and the uppermost layer of the dermis. With deep resurfacing, more of the dermis is removed. Generally, laser resurfacing costs $1,330, on average, for a partial face peel, and $2,700 for full-face resurfacing, according to the American Society of Plastic Surgeons.

Compared with chemical peels, laser resurfacing may offer several advantages. First, the surgeon can more precisely control the depth of the peel. Second, there is little bleeding, if any, and less swelling, bruising, and discomfort following the procedure. And third, recovery time is generally faster—about five to 10 days, on average.

The type of laser used makes a difference in the results and length of recovery. There are approximately nine different types of lasers in use, but two are the most common. The ultrapulsed carbon-dioxide laser, which is highly accurate, gives the best results because it peels away more layers of skin. However, postoperative redness is more severe and can linger for up to three months. For lighter laser peels and a faster recover, the erbium YAG laser is preferable because it is gentler, there is less heat exchange, and the healing time is just three to six weeks.

Some surgeons use both types of lasers during the procedure. Here's why: The ultrapulsed carbon-dioxide laser is ideally suited for treating deeper wrinkles, while the erbium YAG works well for the thinner skin around the eyes.

Another laser being used for resurfacing is the Cool Touch Laser. Together with a cooling spray applied to the skin's surface, this treatment employs an infrared laser passed over the skin. Unlike conventional laser resurfacing, the outer layers of skin are not removed. The laser energy is converted into heat in the dermis in order to stimulate fibroblasts to start generating new collagen. As collagen thickens, the texture and resilience of your skin improves.

Are You a Good Candidate for Laser Resurfacing?

If your skin is olive, brown, or black, this procedure may not be an appropriate option because a laser peel, like most resurfacing operations, can permanently lighten skin, or bring about discoloration. A cosmetic surgeon can evaluate your skin and skin color and decide whether you should undergo the procedure.

Also, if you have taken the retinoid Accutane in the past 12 to 18 months, are prone to scarring, or have a active skin infection, laser resurfacing is not advisable.

Prior to Treatment

Based on your medical history, your cosmetic surgeon will evaluate whether you are a good candidate for laser resurfacing. If the procedure is a go, your surgeon will perform a routine medical examination and photograph your face. He or she may suggest that you use topical tretinoin (Renova or Retin-A) for at least six weeks prior to treatment. Two other treatments may be added to this regimen: hydroquinone cream if you're at risk of skin-color changes following treatment and antiviral medication if you have a history of herpes simplex.

Make arrangements for someone to drive you home following the operation, since you may be in pain or feel groggy from the anesthesia or sedative.

During Treatment

Laser resurfacing is generally performed on an outpatient basis—at an outpatient surgery center or in the physician's office-based facility.

In most cases, a topical anesthetic will be rubbed into your skin to numb the pain during the operation. You may also be given a sedative for relaxation. During the operation, you'll be awake and relaxed, but you won't feel much discomfort. For more extensive laser peels, such as full-face resurfacing, your surgeon may give you a general anesthetic and quite possibly intravenous sedation. In that case, you'll be asleep through the operation.

Next, your skin will be washed with a nonalcohol cleanser. Areas with hair will be covered with wet drapes, and protective eye shields will be placed over your eyes.

During the procedure, the surgeon passes the activated laser over your skin. After the first pass, the treated epidermis is wiped off with a saline-soaked gauze. Next, a dry gauze will absorb any residual water prior to the next pass. Additional passes are made until the wrinkle or scar is less noticeable. Usually, only one or two passes are made around the eyes, and two or three passes are made over other areas.

After your skin has been resurfaced, the surgeon will apply a protective ointment, and in some cases, a bandage, to aid in healing. Your skin may burn a little, but this can be soothed with a cold compress or mild pain reliever.

After Treatment

You may experience some swelling and discomfort, both of which can be controlled with cool water compresses and pain relievers. If a bandage was applied, you should change it the following day and keep it on for several days, or according to your surgeon's instructions. After a week, your surgeon may instruct you to apply a special ointment to the treated skin.

As a normal part of the healing process, your skin may begin to crust. Do not pick the crusts off or you may increase the likelihood of scarring. Crusts usually disappear after about ten days.

Resurfaced skin will be pink or red in the weeks following the operation. This is a result of the new skin that is emerging. Sometimes, though, the redness may last up to six months. Your surgeon may prescribe a medication to reduce the redness.

Usually, you can resume wearing makeup about two weeks following the operation. If your skin is red, try using a makeup with a green cosmetic foundation to conceal the redness.

Once your skin has healed and the color returns to normal, your surgeon may recommend that you resume using tretinoin. If there is some skin discoloration, a hydroquinone cream may be prescribed, too.

Your skin will be quite vulnerable to the damaging effects of sunlight. Using a sunscreen with an SPF of 15 or higher and appropriate sun-blocking clothes will protect your skin from sun damage and help you maintain the results of your laser peel.

The cosmetic results of laser resurfacing are not instantaneous. In fact, it may take several months before your skin begins to take on its new, more youthful glow. The rejuvenating effects of laser resurfacing are not permanent, either, but can last up to five years with proper skin-care management.

Side Effects

As noted above, the most common side effect is skin redness, which gradually disappears. Skin discoloration occurs in about a third of patients undergoing laser resurfacing, but this can be minimized with the use of hydroquinone. The risk of scarring, as well as skin discoloration, is higher with deeper laser peels.

If you have persistent pain, or if the treated area looks infected, see your surgeon immediately.

ELECTROSURGICAL RESURFACING

The latest development in facial rejuvenation is electrosurgical resurfacing. Rather than use heat as lasers do, this technique delivers a high-frequency electrical current to particles in salt water that has been applied to the skin, causing layers of skin to separate and fall off. This approach removes unwanted skin, tightens the skin, and reduces wrinkles. Even though it penetrates as deeply as a laser peel, electrosurgical resurfacing may minimize skin damage and other side effects that are more common with other forms of resurfacing, plus permit a speedier recovery time.

In a news release issued by the American Academy of Dermatology (AAD), dermatologist Tina S. Alster, M.D., said, "Electrosurgical resurfacing is ideal for patients in their 20s, 30s, and 40s, with mild to moderate skin damage and wrinkles, especially around the mouth and eyes. Due to its precision, electrosurgical resurfacing may also be a good choice for scar revision."

Another advantage, according to the AAD, is that it can

be used on all skin types. Traditionally, people with darker skin have not been good candidates for resurfacing because the procedures can permanently alter skin pigment. Electrosurgical resurfacing, however, does not affect the skin's pigment.

A study conducted by Alastair Carruthers, M.D., the first person to use electrosurgical resurfacing on human skin, found that the technology produced a reasonable result on crow's-feet six months after treatment.

Typically, electrosurgical skin resurfacing takes 30 to 60 minutes. It is significantly less painful than other resurfacing techniques. Immediately afterward your skin will appear pink and be slightly swollen, a condition that lasts for a few days. But within a week, these side effects will subside, and you can resume wearing makeup. After two weeks, all redness will disappear. Like other forms of laser resurfacing, this method can activate herpes simplex lesions.

PULSED-LIGHT THERAPY

One of the newest skin resurfacing technologies is *intense pulsed-light therapy,* which can erase fine lines and wrinkles, plus smooth out other skin imperfections. Instead of a laser, it employs multiple wavelengths of light sent through the skin. The light generates heat and, in the process, stimulates dermal cells to produce more collagen. Research indicates that collagen production may increase by as much as 20 percent.

The procedure takes about 45 minutes, and there are virtually no side effects. You can put makeup on afterward and return to work immediately. Normally, six treatments are required to delete wrinkles and other skin flaws. A series of six treatments costs approximately $2,000.

If you are interested in exploring pulsed-light therapy or

any other resurfacing procedure, consult a cosmetic surgeon who is knowledgeable and experienced in performing the procedure. A good source of information is the American Society of Plastic Surgeons. You can locate qualified surgeons by accessing the organization's Web site at www.plasticsurgery.org.

13

The Age-Stopping Face-lift

I N the United States, the face-lift ranks among the top five most popular cosmetic surgeries, with nearly 75,000 performed annually, according to the American Society of Plastic Surgeons (ASPS). Technically known as *rhytidectomy,* a face-lift makes you look younger by removing and tightening excess skin and fat. The procedure removes deeper, coarser wrinkles, and gives your skin a smoother appearance. A face-lift is often performed in conjunction with other cosmetic surgeries, such as eyelid surgery or a forehead lift, and outer-skin-rejuvenation procedures like chemical peels or laser resurfacing.

The cost of a face-lift varies widely, depending on the surgeon, the extent of the face-lift, and the area of the country in which you live, but a typical face-lift costs about $5,000. Because it is considered elective surgery, a face-lift is not normally covered by health insurance.

ARE YOU A GOOD CANDIDATE
FOR A FACE-LIFT?

Face-lifts are performed mostly on women 51 to 64 years old, although the procedure can be done on people in their seventies and eighties. You're an ideal candidate if the skin on your face and neck has begun to droop, but still retains some elasticity, and your facial bone structure is strong.

Your medical history and health habits also determine whether you're a good candidate for a face-lift. Generally, the healthier you are, the better the face-lift will go. By contrast, certain habits can adversely affect the procedure, including a history of drug abuse and alcoholism. If obese, you may be a poor candidate, too, because only some of the fat can be taken out, and you may not like the results.

Other poor candidates are those with dark skin, since scarring may be more apparent.

REALISTIC EXPECTATIONS

If considering a face-lift, approach it realistically. Foremost, keep in mind that this type of surgery can't make you look like you did in your twenties.

"For instance, the notion that a face lift will make one look '10 years younger' is likely to be overly optimistic," cautioned B. J. Landis, Ph.D., in *The Nurse Practitioner.* "It may be more accurate to say it makes one 'look good for their age.'"

Dr. Landis also noted: "In most cases, facial cosmetic surgery has a positive impact and builds one's self-esteem."

To show you what a face-lift might do for you, your surgeon may have you lie on your back and look upward into a mirror. In that position, your skin gravitates downward and appears temporarily tighter.

Some cosmetic surgeons employ imaging devices and special computer software to demonstrate how a face-lift might improve your appearance.

FINDING A QUALIFIED SURGEON

If you are seriously considering a face-lift, it is vital to consult an experienced, reputable surgeon. The final results of your face-lift depend largely on the skill of the surgeon you select. He or she should be uniquely qualified to perform this procedure and experienced in the field of plastic surgery. What's more, a surgeon should be an artist of sorts—someone who knows how to design and plan a procedure according to your own unique facial characteristics.

To find a surgeon with this blend of medical expertise and artistry, here are some important guidelines:

◊ Research and verify the surgeon's credentials. Your surgeon should be board certified in plastic surgery. Other good sources of information about surgeons include your city, county, and state medical societies; your personal physician; and the Better Business Bureau.

◊ Find out how many procedures a surgeon has performed.

◊ Ask to see before and after photographs of patients, or better yet, talk to former patients. A surgeon should have an artistic ability.

◊ Find out what the costs will be.

◊ Ask to see complication rates—the percentage of patients who have experienced complications and side effects following surgery.

Finally, make sure you feel comfortable with the surgeon, and do not go through with the face-lift unless you do.

Prior to Surgery

Once your surgeon has determined you're an appropriate candidate for a face-lift, he or she will evaluate your face and discuss your goals and expectations for the operation. During this consultation, you'll have routine blood tests, go over any allergies and medical conditions with your surgeon, review the surgical plan, get answers to any last-minute questions, and sign consents.

In addition, your surgeon will probably ask you about any medications you're taking. Aspirin, alcohol, warfarin (Coumadin), vitamin E, and vitamin E–containing products may increase bleeding during surgery. Thus it's wise to avoid these products for a few weeks prior to your operation. If you smoke, you should quit a week or two prior to surgery, because smoking thwarts blood flow to the skin and will interfere with healing.

In addition, if you have short hair, your surgeon may recommend that you grow it longer to hide postsurgery scars while they heal.

During Surgery

A face-lift is performed under general anesthesia and as an outpatient operation. In some cases, the surgeon will administer local anesthesia and a sedative. The entire procedure will take several hours.

In a standard face-lift operation, the surgeon makes incisions in the hairline at the temples, in front of the ear, and behind the earlobe to the lower scalp. Next, the skin is lifted and separated from the muscle and bones below. Excess skin is trimmed, and fat may be removed from around the neck and chin to enhance the coutours of your face. The surgeon redrapes the skin across your face and reattaches it to the incisions around the hairline and ear.

Staples or metal clips are used to close the scalp incisions. The net effect is tightening and smoothing of facial skin.

To prevent fluid buildup after surgery, drains in the form of small thin tubes are usually placed beneath the skin under the ears and along the suture lines.

After Surgery

Your face will be bandaged, and the bandages must remain in place from at least 24 hours to five days. Expect to experience temporary bruising and swelling. Your skin will feel tender, dry, and tight in some places. Keep your head elevated, and apply cold compresses to minimize swelling or bleeding.

The day after surgery, your surgeon will remove the drains and examine your incisions. You may experience pain for several days after the operation, but this can be relieved with painkillers.

You'll be given a written, detailed set of postoperative instructions on alcohol avoidance, sleep and posture (there is less tendency to bleed if you keep your head elevated), sexual activity, shampooing, bathing, and general activity. You should follow these instructions to the letter to avoid complications and enhance the healing process.

Two weeks following your surgery, your surgeon will remove the staples. Your cheek and neck areas may feel numb; however, sensation will gradually return. To prevent burns, don't use hair dryers or curling irons until the feeling comes back. Your face will also be puffy.

About 48 hours following your surgery, you can resume a normal routine. Most patients, however, take three or four weeks off from work in order to recover. You may have bruising and discoloration for about a month. Don't pursue any strenuous sports for at least a month, and limit your sun exposure for several months.

Complications and Side Effects

A face-lift, like any surgical procedure, is not without risks and complications. It's critical to understand what they are, so make sure your surgeon thoroughly discusses them with you. What follows is a brief description of potential complications. Your surgeon should fill you in on others.

Infection. Although extremely rare, infection may occur. It can be easily treated with antibiotics. Signs of infection include localized heat, redness, and pain. If you notice any of these signs at or near the incision areas, notify your surgeon immediately.

Scarring. The areas of incision will leave slight scars, but these can be concealed by your hair. Scars fade with time and will become less noticeable.

Permanent Loss of Sensation. Incisions made on the scalp may cut nerves, resulting in the loss of sensation. This has been known to occur in a nerve near the ear, in particular, and may result in permanent numbness of the earlobe. But as noted above, most loss of sensation reverses itself in a few months. There may also be injury to the nerves that control your facial muscles, but this side effect is usually temporary.

Hematoma. This is a collection of blood that forms under the skin. It must be surgically removed by your surgeon. Hematoma occurs in about 2 percent of all cases and shows up usually in the first few hours following the operation.

Hair loss. You may experience some hair loss around the scars.

Psychological Complications. Following surgery, some women become depressed because they are dissatisfied with the results. This can be averted, however, if you're fully informed about what to expect during recovery and have realistic expectations about what a face-lift will do for your looks.

OTHER SURGICAL PROCEDURES FOR FACIAL REJUVENATION

Since 1992, the number of cosmetic-surgery procedures among women has jumped by a whopping 165 percent, according to a recent report from the American Society of Plastic Surgeons.

"Cosmetic surgery is more popular than ever," noted the Society's president, C. Lin Puckett, M.D. "Both women and men are choosing cosmetic procedures to keep their youthful appearance and feel good about themselves. Also, the technical advancements made in plastic surgery over the last few years have made cosmetic procedures easier and safer for the patient."

Among the many cosmetic procedures growing in popularity is eyelid surgery ("blepharoplasty"), which corrects drooping eyelids and puffy bags under eyes—two conditions that make you look older. More than 140,000 eyelid surgeries are performed annually, and that number is on the rise, particularly among women. For both eyelids, the surgery costs approximately $3,000. It involves removing fat and excessive skin from the upper and lower lids.

Performed under local anesthesia, eyelid surgery takes one to three hours, depending on the extent of the operation. The surgeon makes tiny incisions in the creases of your upper lids and just below your eyelashes in your lower lids. Underlying fat and extra skin is removed, and the incisions are closed with small sutures.

You'll have bruising and swelling following surgery, but they will subside in two weeks to a month. As with a face-lift, you must follow your surgeon's postoperative instructions very closely.

The risks associated with eyelid surgery include infection, reaction to anesthesia, temporary blurred or double vision, and swelling of the eyelids. You should not undergo eyelid surgery if you suffer from thyroid disease, dry eye, high blood pressure, circulatory disorders, heart disease, or diabetes.

Another cosmetic procedure that restores a youthful appearance to your face is a forehead lift, also called a brow lift. With age, your upper facial structure begins to droop. Forehead lifts correct this, plus remove horizontal wrinkles on the forehead. The procedure costs about $2,500, on average. It is often performed in conjunction with eyelid surgery.

In a forehead lift, the surgeon makes incisions along the hairline and the frontal scalp hairline, following a "headphone-type pattern." The skin of your forehead is then lifted so that the underlying muscle can be altered or removed. This tends to smooth out the overlying skin. The incisions are closed with stitches or staples.

Increasingly, forehead lifts are being performed with a viewing instrument called an *endoscope*. This lets the surgeon make only three to five tiny incisions rather than one long incision at the hairline. With this technique, the surgeon uses a very small scope, along with a camera that magnifies the surgical area, to view the muscles and tissues under the skin. Using another instrument, the surgeon lifts the skin and makes the necessary alterations to the tissue underneath.

After the operation, you'll experience swelling, discomfort, and itching around the incision and possibly a minor headache. Follow your surgeon's instructions for postoperative care to enhance the healing process.

Though rare, complications may include paralysis of the nerves that control eyebrow movement; scar formation;

hair loss along the scar edges; and temporary loss of sensation near the incisions.

People who undergo forehead lifts are usually pleased with the dramatic improvement the operation makes in their appearance. Even though the results last many years, you may want to have another forehead lift at some point in the future.

A MORE YOUTHFUL LOOK

Even though you've had a face-lift or other facial cosmetic procedure, your face will continue to age. That being so, you must continue to take good care of your complexion with nonsurgical approaches, such as tretinoin, hydroxy acids, moisturizers, liberal use of sunscreen, or other methods recommended by your dermatologist or cosmetic surgeon. The younger-looking benefits of a facial cosmetic surgery generally last around five to 10 years. Thus it's conceivable that you may want to have another face-lift at some point in the future so that you can continue to look more youthful.

PART SIX

Skin Management for Life

14

Wrinkle-Reducing Makeup

OUT of a bottle, tube, or jar come the finishing touches to your antiwrinkle program: makeup. It has the power to conceal wrinkles, perfect your complexion, and make you look younger in a matter of minutes.

There's more: Besides revitalizing your face, makeup has plenty of other benefits, according to scientific studies. A growing body of research shows that wearing makeup:

◊ Enhances others' perception of you.

◊ Strengthens your self-image.

◊ Makes you feel more socially secure.

◊ Lifts your mood during bouts of depression.

◊ Produces a more positive outlook on life.

There's even an economic impact of wearing makeup: You can make more money! One study discovered that women of all age groups (including those over 65) could substantially increase their salaries by wearing appropriately applied makeup.

What's more, *cosmetic therapy*—the use of makeup as a therapeutic technique to help ease the suffering of people who have been facially disfigured—is now widely accepted as a submedical specialty in dermatology and cosmetic surgery. Writing in *Dermatologic Clinics,* Marvin G. Westmore, a medical makeup specialist, noted: "The timely use of makeup in the rehabilitation of patients promotes psychologic well-being, higher self-esteem, and greater social acceptance by society."

Clearly, there's more to makeup than meets the eye!

ANTIAGING MAKEUP

Let's face it: We're not all as young as we'd like to be. Even so, the next best thing to being young is looking young. And that's where makeup comes in.

There are three broad categories of makeup: fashion makeup, camouflage makeup, and theatrical makeup. You may opt to use one of these, or a combination. When applied properly, they are useful for masking wrinkles, age spots, and other signs of aging. Here are the basics.

FASHION MAKEUP

Quite probably, you already use *fashion makeup,* which is sold in pharmacies, department-store cosmetics counters, and other retail outlets. These products include foundations, concealers, powders, blushes, rouges, eyeliners, eyebrow pencils, eye shadows, mascara, lipsticks, and lip glosses.

For mature skin, a most recent innovation in fashion makeup is light-diffusing makeup. It contains tiny particles (usually mica) or pigments that reflect and redirect light from your face so that wrinkles and fine lines are less noticeable. Examples of light-diffusing foundations are Lancôme Photogenic Skin-Illuminating Makeup SPF 15, Prescriptions' Luxe Soft Glow Moisture Makeup, L'Oréal Visuelle Invisible Coverage Makeup, and Elizabeth Arden's Flawless Finish Hydro Light Foundation.

Light-diffusing foundation is not to be confused with shimmer makeup—products that contain silvery golden flecks and make your skin look sparkly. Leave the shimmery stiff to teenagers and twenty-somethings, since it only makes wrinkles more pronounced.

Another antiaging formulation is Revlon's Age-Defying Liquid Makeup. Available in sixteen shades, this foundation contains moisturizer-wrapped color particles that float above fine facial lines to help hide them.

An Internet company called AFE Cosmetics and Skincare offers custom-blend foundations for all skin types, including mature skin. Using an on-line or mail-in order form, you select the qualities you want in a foundation. Options include oil-free, enriched, extra moisture, liquid, sheer, or extra coverage. You can also opt to have color correctors or luminizers blended into the foundation. The company takes that information and customizes makeup just for you. I have purchased makeup from AFE Cosmetics and Skincare and have found its foundation to be excellent for concealing wrinkles. The Internet address is www.cosmetics.com.

Fashion makeup is often formulated with other ingredients that are beneficial to aging skin. These include moisturizers to prevent water loss, sunscreens to block harmful ultraviolet rays, and antioxidants to guard against free-radical damage to your skin. If you need these additional protective factors, then a foundation containing them is a good choice for your skin.

CAMOUFLAGE MAKEUP

Camouflage makeup is designed to downplay facial defects, normalize appearance, and accentuate the more attractive features of your face. It is used primarily in dermatology and plastic surgery to hide acne scars, traumatic scars, disease-caused skin discolorations, veins, and other skin problems. But it also does an admirable job of concealing wrinkles.

In addition, camouflage makeup can be applied following a chemical peel, laser resurfacing, filler procedures, or a face-lift to conceal temporary aftereffects such as redness, bruising, swelling, or visible injection or incision marks. It is initially applied by a qualified medical camouflage therapist, who, in turn, teaches patients how to apply the makeup themselves.

If you're preparing to undergo a cosmetic facial procedure, be sure to meet with a camouflage therapist beforehand. The therapist will select the right makeup for you, based on your lifestyle, cosmetic preferences, and budget, and teach you how to apply it. You'll learn how to disguise incision lines and bruises; correct for color in case your skin is red in places; and contour to hide swelling by creating the illusion of highlights and shadows.

"When the patients no longer see the post-surgical redness, bruising and/or scars, and a beautiful makeup is applied, you can see the relief in their faces," wrote Nancy Ogden-West in *Skin Pharmacology and Applied Skin Physiology.* "They feel more attractive again, and they start to have a great appreciation for the surgery they have just gone through." Ogden-West is coordinator of the Skin Enhancement Center in Mayfield Heights, Ohio.

During your meeting, the therapist will want to know about:

◊ Your participation in sports or outdoor activities (the makeup must fit your lifestyle).

◊ Your work environment, particularly its lighting. That way, the therapist can select makeup that will look the best under certain lighting conditions.

◊ Sensitivities you have to certain cosmetics.

◊ Skin-care products you're currently using.

◊ Your economic situation (in order to select makeup you can reasonably afford).

These and other considerations help create the optimum cosmetic treatment plan following cosmetic procedures, plus help you look your very best during the recovery period.

There are a variety of camouflage cosmetics available, including foundations, color correctors, and rouges. Compared with traditional fashion makeup, camouflage makeup is more opaque, thicker, more water resistant, and longer-lasting, providing eight hours or more of wear. What's more, it is formulated to adhere to scar tissue without coming off.

You can purchase camouflage makeup directly from numerous manufacturers. One of these is Covermark Cosmetics, founded more than 60 years ago by Lydia O'Leary, who was born with a port-wine-stain birthmark that covered her face. In the 1930s, O'Leary was unable to get a job because of this facial disfigurement. Knowledgeable in chemistry and painting, she developed and marketed her own concealment makeup. It is the only makeup foundation that has ever been granted a U.S. patent.

Today, Covermark Cosmetics sells an extensive line of cosmetics. Facial products include Classic Covermark, for concealing serious skin flaws; Face Magic, a creamy foundation designed to hide undereye circles, age spots, and acne; and Coverstik, a concealer. All of these products are available in numerous shades. You can purchase them online at www.covermark.com.

Sold at JCPenney and other fine department stores, Dermablend Corrective Cosmetics were developed for physicians to camouflage imperfections such as acne scarring, burns, veins, pigment changes, and other skin problems. Dermablend cosmetics for the face include Dermablend Cover Crème, a fragrance-free foundation that is long-lasting and provides superior coverage without being heavy; Dermablend Setting Powder, designed to be applied over the Cover Crème; Quick-Fix Concealer, for hiding small facial flaws; and Wrinkle-Fix, a moisturizing treatment for lip and eye areas. There is also a bronzer to add a natural-looking contour to your complexion.

More than 60 years ago, an allergist, Dr. Frank Crandall, created a line of makeup called Physicians Formula for his wife, who had sensitive skin. Today, Physicians Formula has expanded to include makeup for mature or damaged skin, postsurgical correction, and the concealment of acne, birthmarks, and other minor skin imperfections. There are a variety of foundations, including a sun-protective (SPF 15) liquid makeup, oil-control matte makeup, light-diffusing makeup, and a light-coverage blend. Several of the foundations are enriched with vitamins A, C, and E. All the products are hypoallergenic, fragrance-free, and dermatologist tested. Physicians Formula products are available in more than 17,000 stores throughout the United States and are distributed in numerous countries worldwide. You can buy Physicians Formula products on-line, too, at www.physiciansformula.com.

Another camouflage product is Veil Cover Cream, formulated in 1952 by a cosmetic chemist, Thomas Blake, to camouflage postoperative scarring. Waterproof and smudgeproof, Veil Cover Cream is used to cover skin blemishes of all types. The product comes in a wide range of skin shades, and there is a translucent powder—Veil Finishing Powder—that helps set the cream. Both are British products, but can be purchased on-line at www.veilcover.com.

Cosmetic giants who manufacture traditional fashion makeup also produce camouflage makeup. Estée Lauder, for example, has a product called Maximum Cover, designed to be used after cosmetic surgery as well as to conceal surgical scars and other skin imperfections. Suitable for all skin types, this makeup is waterproof and has an SPF of 15. I have tried this foundation and can attest to its benefits. It feels velvety when applied and is long-lasting. The coverage by the end of the day is as smooth and as even as when it was first applied in the morning.

Clinique's Continuous Coverage foundation features an opaque formulation to cover birthmarks, scars, and other skin flaws. It can be used as a concealer or as full-face makeup. Available in five shades, Continuous Coverage contains a sunblock and has an SPF of 11. I have tried this foundation, too. It provides excellent coverage and long wear, plus it makes your skin look very smooth.

Lancôme offers a full-coverage product called Dual Finish that doubles as a foundation and a powder. It imparts a matte finish and is suitable for all skin types. There are 16 different shades.

THEATRICAL MAKEUP

In the strictest sense, *theatrical makeup* is used primarily in the entertainment industry to glamorize actors, television stars, and other performers, or help them meet the cosmetic requirements of their various roles. Theatrical makeup is both corrective and creative.

As a corrective product, it conceals blemishes and other skin flaws, imparts a smooth look and even skin tone for photography and lighting, helps define facial features, and makes the performer look more attractive. As a creative product, theatrical makeup is used to change the look of performers, making them appear younger or older, giving them scars or wounds, or transforming them into extraterrestrials.

Theatrical makeup—also known as grease paint—is also employed in dermatology and cosmetic surgery to conceal or fill in scars and other facial defects because it is thick, waxy, and very long-lasting.

Pancake makeup is a well-known form of theatrical makeup used in dermatology and cosmetic surgery because it does an excellent job of covering and hiding facial defects. It was developed in the thirties by Max Factor, Sr., a renowned Hollywood makeup artist, to solve the makeup problems created by the introduction of Technicolor to movies. (The makeup used in black-and-white films didn't translate well to color films; it would make actors' faces look green or red.)

Packaged in a flat, rounded container, pancake makeup is a solid material that contains talc, titanium dioxide, various oxides, and chalk, among other ingredients. Applied with a moist sponge, it provides a matte finish, which tends to camouflage wrinkles well. Pancake makeup continues to be one of the most popular forms of makeup worldwide.

Generally, theatrical makeup is sold directly to the entertainment industry and to medical cosmetic professionals through a number of retailers and wholesalers. If you are interested in experimenting with theatrical makeup, look for the following brands: Cinema Secrets, Ben Nye Company, Inc., Marvin Westmore Cosmetics, and Joe Blasco Cosmetics. These are also sold through various Web sites.

FACE-SAVING APPLICATION TECHNIQUES

There's a lot to the use of makeup to hide the appearance of wrinkles, blemishes, and other marks of aging, so let's take it step-by-step.

Step 1: Use a Neutralizer

The first step is to apply a *neutralizer,* particularly if your face has blemishes, discolorations, or other minor imperfections. Neutralizers have been around since the twenties and are worn underneath your foundation. They are available as liquids or creams and contain special compensating tints.

Green neutralizers conceal redness; lavender counterbalances yellowish areas of skin; brown corrects white scars; orange or peach offsets the black-and-blue of bruises; and white neutralizers are excellent for downplaying wrinkles and dark areas.

After the neutralizer is applied to the affected areas, it should be set with powder, followed by an application of foundation.

Step 2: Apply Your Foundation

Foundations are generally available as *light coverage, medium or moderate coverage,* and *heavy, full, maximum, or extra coverage.* These designations describe how thickly or thinly the product coats the skin once it is applied. Most camouflage or theatrical foundations are of the heavy or full-coverage variety. They contain a high concentration of titanium oxide, a sunblock that promotes better coverage.

Among cosmetic experts, there is some disagreement as to which coverage is best for aging skin. Most advise moderate to full coverage because these preparations do a better job of concealing fine lines and wrinkles. On the other hand, proponents of light-coverage makeup believe that it evens out mature skin, without appearing too masklike, and is less likely to settle in the folds of wrinkles.

The bottom line is that you'll have to experiment with different types of coverage. If you find that your foundation pools in wrinkles—a problem that makes wrinkles more apparent—then it's time to switch to a different product. Personally, I've found that heavy or full-coverage foundations do a better job of hiding wrinkles and are longer-lasting.

Foundations are sold as liquids, creams, or pancake. Again, you have to "test-drive" which type best suits your skin. Liquid makeup tends to provide lighter coverage; creams and pancake makeup, moderate to heavy coverage.

Foundations come in the following formulations: oil-free; water-in-oil, which contains a higher concentration of water; and oil-in-water, which has less water. Heavy-coverage foundations generally contain more oil. If your skin is on the oily side, choose an oil-free product. Dry-skin types do better with oil-in-water formulas.

The right shade of foundation is important, too. Go too light, and your skin will look unnaturally pale and washed out; too dark, and you'll be able to see where your foundation ends and your natural skin color begins (usually at the jawline or upper neckline).

Most foundations come in a variety of pigments so that your natural skin tone can be accurately matched. Test shades out by blending them, one at a time, into your neck or jawbone. Then view them in natural light. The shade that best matches your natural skin color is the right choice. When shopping for makeup on-line, you'll have to wing it and select the color sample that most closely approximates your skin color.

In addition, cosmetic experts feel that pink- or peach-tone foundations make you look older. In some cases, you must blend various shades of foundation to come up with the perfect match for your skin color.

To apply the foundation, gently dab the makeup on your skin, beginning in the central part of your face and blending outward until you smooth it over your entire face. Use a disposable makeup sponge or your fingertips. Be sure to blend it into your hairline slightly and under your chin for a more natural appearance. Applying foundation on your neck can call attention to wrinkles.

Step 3: Touch Up with Concealers

Concealers are handy tools for spot-treating and covering up dark spots (such as those under the eyes), hiding blemishes, and filling in crow's-feet and marionette lines. Generally, you should use a concealer that matches your skin color. If you have dark undereye circles, however, use a concealer that's one shade lighter than your skin and smooth it over those dark areas.

Concealers are available in various forms and consistencies. Sticks, which tend to be heavier, are excellent for spot touch-ups such as pimples. They work well if your skin is normal to oily.

Concealers that come in pots are creamier and thicker and provide more concentrated coverage over large areas. They are appropriate for drier skin.

Pencil-type concealers are great for covering tiny spots or fine lines. Plus, they resist caking. Some pencil concealers are designed specifically for disguising wrinkles.

Other concealers come in tubes. Lighter and easy to apply, these products work best on normal to dry skin.

To apply a concealer, gently pat it on your skin with your little finger. No matter which concealer you use, it's best to apply it on top of your regular foundation and before you powder your face.

Step 4: Set Your Foundation with Powder

Facial powder sets your foundation and gives your face a finished, more youthful look. In addition, powder prevents smudging and makes your foundation last longer. Translucent face powder is preferable for mature skin because it gives the complexion a more even finish. Most camouflage foundations are designed to be worn with powder.

After applying the neutralizer, foundation, and concealer, wait about five minutes before powdering. Then press—do not dust—the powder on top of the foundation. Wait a few minutes for the powder to set, then brush off any excess. Powder tends to accumulate in fine lines and can magnify them. (If your powder looks like it has collected in wrinkles, its granules are probably not fine enough. Switch brands.)

There are many types of powders on the market. Loose powder is perfect for reducing shine (which intensifies wrinkles and other imperfections). So are oil-control powders, which contain oil-absorbing silica. For dry skin, try a pressed powder because it is higher in oil. Pressed powders provide heavier coverage.

For minimizing wrinkles, you might opt for a light-diffusing product. Among the light-diffusing powders on the market are Estée Lauder's Lucidity Translucent Powder and Almay's Time-off Age Smoothing Pressed Powder.

Step 5: Apply Lipstick

Lipstick is the one cosmetic women will not leave home without wearing, according to a Revlon-commissioned survey of 400 women between the ages 45 and 65. So when you do put it on, make sure you do so correctly.

Lipstick is tricky, with a penchant for wandering into areas where it shouldn't be—such as into those tiny vertical lines that run perpendicular to the mouth.

Here's how to keep lip color from straying:

First, apply foundation over your lips before putting on lipstick. Then line your lips with a lip pencil as a kind of hedge. The wax in the lip pencil prevents lipstick from bleeding.

Matte-finish lipsticks are drier and stay in place better. But if you have dry or chapped lips, try a moisturizing lipstick instead.

If you have vertical lines above your upper lips, select a light shade of lipstick. That way, if it bleeds, it won't be so visible.

Step 6: Apply the Finishing Touches

These include blushes, eye shadow, mascara, and eyeliners. Blushes give a hint of color to cheeks and can help contour your face. It's best to use a powdered blush because it adheres better to the foundation. A blush that is too orange may make you look older. So will sparkly or frosty blushes. Brushing in an upward motion, apply blush to the upper part of your cheek.

Generally, powdered eye shadows last longer than cream-based products. Avoid using sparkly or frosty shadows, since they exaggerate the crinkled eyelids of mature skin.

To accentuate your eyes, apply a light-colored shadow to the upper eyelid and a slightly darker shade of the same color to the lower part of the eyelid. Light neutral shades such as beiges, taupe, light browns, or plums work best. No bright colors—they only call attention to droopy eyelids and wrinkled skin.

Eyelids do sag with age. To give them an illusory lift, define the upper lids with a very thin line of liquid eyeliner. Or apply a pencil liner and smudge it a bit on upper and lower lids. Then curl your eyelashes upward to give your eyes a lifted look.

As for mascara, lengthen your upper lashes with plenty of coats. But go light on your lower lashes to de-emphasize undereye circles and bags. Use a color that best approximates that of your natural color. Stay away from colored mascara, since it looks too artificial and may call unwanted attention to marks of aging around your eyes.

LOOKING YOUR BEST

To hide your age-related flaws and bring out your best, you may have to try different brands of makeup. A good test of makeup is to check it after eight hours of wear: If it remains in place and doesn't accumulate in fine lines and wrinkles (especially those under and around the eyes), then it's the best makeup for you.

15
Your Personal Skin-Rejuvenation Program

THERE'S no denying it: Your face is the most exposed part of your body and is under constant assault from the environment as well as from the natural forces of aging that seem to get stronger with each passing year. Maintaining a luminous, younger-looking complexion can be a challenge.

The question is: What should you be doing, starting now, to turn back the hands of time, or at least slow them down?

Answer: It depends largely on the present condition of your complexion and its degree of wrinkling. No two women have exactly the same skin or skin problems. But as you've learned in this book, there are products, treatments, and procedures designed for practically every situation. You have to choose what's best for you, and in many cases, your dermatologist can assist. In addition, this chapter will help you design a skin-rejuvenation program that will lead to a much-improved complexion.

But first: There are several basic actions everyone should take, regardless of age or skin condition, to prevent

wrinkles, slow down their formation, and promote good
skin health in general. Let's take a look.

FOLLOW A SKIN-HEALTHY LIFESTYLE

What skin needs is a healthy lifestyle. That involves diet,
exercise, no smoking, and stress management.

A skin-healthy diet is one that's rich in fruits, vegetables, and whole grains. These foods contain antioxidants,
which fight free radicals, unstable oxygen molecules that
attack bodily tissues, including skin.

"Wrinkling, which is accelerated by sun exposure, occurs as a result of oxidative damage," noted dermatologist
Alan M. Dattner, M.D., in an interview in the *Journal of
Women's Health & Gender-Based Medicine.* "It stands to
reason that a diet rich in antioxidants can help promote
healthy skin by protecting it from free radical-environ-
mental stresses."

Thus, fortify your skin nutritionally, starting with meals.
Make sure you eat at least five servings of fruits and vegetables daily, and with every meal, some protein (fish,
poultry, lean meats, legumes, or low-fat dairy products).
Include several servings of whole grains daily, too.

To ensure sufficient antioxidant intake and protection
from free radicals, it is wise to take a once-a-day vita-
min/mineral tablet containing antioxidant nutrients. You
may also want to consider supplementing with more vitamin C and vitamin E than can be found in a multiple vita-
min/mineral supplement.

Based on available evidence on antioxidants, here are
suggested daily intakes from food and supplements:

◊ 10,000 to 20,000 International Units of beta-
    carotene

◊ 400 to 800 International Units of vitamin E

◊ 200 to 500 milligrams of vitamin C

◊ Up to 50 micrograms of selenium

◊ 2 milligrams of copper

◊ 12 milligrams of zinc

◊ Up to 5 milligrams of manganese

Other nutritional supplements that may help your skin are evening primrose oil and borage oil. Both contain essential fatty acids (EFAs), which, among other duties, keep your skin smooth. That's because they are loaded with gamma-linolenic acid, a nutrient that has a hand in promoting healthy skin, hair, and nails. In clinical trials, evening primrose oil has been shown to reduce the severity of eczema, an inflammation of the skin that produces dryness, scaliness, and itching. Many alternative health-care practitioners recommend taking 500 milligrams of one of these supplements each day. You should notice an improvement in your skin in about six to eight weeks.

Drinking at least eight to 10 glasses of water daily is another skin-healthy habit. When skin is well hydrated, it's less likely to become dry and wrinkly. You can easily test your skin's level of hydration. With your fingers, pull up a bit of skin on the back of one hand, then let go. If the skin quickly retracts into place, you're well hydrated. But if it stays momentarily in a tentlike position, you need more water.

Regular exercise is important, too, because it increases circulation to the skin. With exercise—particularly the heart-pumping aerobic type—your capillaries increase in size and number, so that more oxygen and nutrients find their way to the skin and other tissues. Your skin gains a healthy glow as a result. Try to exercise at least 30 minutes a day, most days of the week.

Over time, smoking makes you look much older than your years by increasing wrinkles and other marks of aging. A major reason behind the aging effects of smoking is that it chokes off oxygen to your skin and other tissues. According to the American Academy of Dermatology, smoking for 10 minutes decreases your body's oxygen supplies for almost an hour; smoking a pack a day significantly interferes with your body's oxygen levels for most of the day. To preserve a youthful look, quit smoking.

Stress gets under your skin. If you're an emotional basket case, do your skin good by getting stress and tension under control. Some stress-management techniques recommended by physicians Michael R. Bilkis, M.D., and Kenneth A. Mark, M.D., in the *Archives of Dermatology* include meditation, affirmation, journal writing, prayer, biofeedback, hypnosis, good nutrition, exercise, and general improvement in lifestyle.

MAKE GOOD SKIN CARE A HABIT

How you treat your skin in the morning and again at night will go a long way toward preserving its precious health and youthfulness. To accomplish that, your skin will thrive on a four-step plan of care.

Wash

For a glowing complexion, you'll need to remove cosmetics, dirt, dead skin cells, and bacteria from your face through regular washing. "Rather than treat the face like a piece of wood that needs to be polished twice a day, women need only wash their faces once daily with warm water and a mild cleanser, using their hands," noted dermatologist Albert M. Kligman, M.D., Ph.D., in the *Journal of Women's Health & Gender-Based Medicine.*

It's best to wash your face in the evening before bedtime. The next morning, simply wash your face with lukewarm water or dab it with a nonalcoholic toner. Many women go to bed with makeup still on—a practice that clogs pores. So always wash your face before retiring.

Most makeup can be washed off with soap and water. Among the products recommended by dermatologists are mild soaps such as Dove, Tone, Caress, Basis, Neutrogena, or a nondrying cleanser like Cetaphil. Foaming gels and cleansers work well, too. There are also exfoliating cleansers formulated with granules that do a good job of sloughing off dead skin cells. If your skin is sensitive or allergy-prone, use a fragrance-free cleanser.

If your makeup is waterproof (many camouflage foundations are), you'll need to use some type of oil-based cleanser to remove it, followed by soap and water for final cleansing. Any residual camouflage makeup can then be swabbed off with an alcohol-free toner applied with a cotton ball.

Be gentle with your skin during cleansing. Scrubbing can irritate skin. Washcloths work best if you have normal to oily skin. With drier skin, use your hands, facial cleansing pads, or an infant's washcloth. Use a slow, upward motion while cleansing.

There's no one cleanser that is perfect for every skin type. You'll have to make some trial runs before deciding on a favorite.

Exfoliate

Exfoliation—the process of sloughing off dead skin cells—helps increase the turnover of epidermal cells and makes your skin look smoother. There are two general types of exfoliation: mechanical and chemical.

Mechanical exfoliants such as washcloths, loofah sponges, and cleansing grains or scrubs work by rubbing and stimulating the surface of the skin. Any of these tools thus cleanses and exfoliates at the same time. A cautionary red flag: Loofah sponges can be a breeding ground for a variety of bacteria because they tend to entrap sloughed-off dead skin cells. Thus, after using a loofah as an exfoliative aid, sterilize it by soaking it in a bleach-and-water solution.

If your skin is delicate or sensitive, be gentle when using mechanical exfoliants because they can redden the skin and possibly cause inflammation. In addition, excessive rubbing can aggravate acne by rupturing whiteheads and increasing inflammation. Skin specialists say that mechanical exfoliation is best if you have a normal or dry skin. You don't need to mechanically exfoliate with every cleansing. For best results, exfoliate no more than three times a week for at least a minute or two.

Chemical exfoliants include hydroxy acids, tretinoin (Renova or Retin-A), and chemical peels. These give your face a fresher appearance by loosening dead skin cells and promoting the growth of new skin cells.

Moisturize

If your skin is normal to dry, moisturizing is a good idea. Moisturizers encourage the skin to retain and hold water, making your complexion look refreshed. They should be applied to damp skin after washing. For more information on moisturizers, see chapter 4.

Protect

Don't leave home without sunscreen applied to your face! It's the best protection you have against wrinkles and should always be worn. Sunscreen is especially important if you exfoliate on a regular basis. Exfoliation makes skin more sun-sensitive because dead skin cells act as sun-protectants. Use a sunscreen with an SPF of 15 or higher or makeup that has at least an SPF of 15.

PERSONALIZED DEFENSE AGAINST WRINKLES

In addition to the guidance discussed above, you'll want to customize your skin-care program according to your age and degree of wrinkling and skin damage.

A word of caution: Other than sunscreen and a moisturizer, do not use more than one topical product at a time, unless your dermatologist has advised otherwise. Many women get so obsessed with treating wrinkles that they use tretinoin, hydroxy acids, coQ10 creams, Kinerase, and other wrinkle creams together. Guess what? You could be aging your skin. The more products you rub on your skin, the greater the risk of irritation and inflammation. Inflammation generates skin-damaging free radicals, which ultimately lead to wrinkles.

One course of action may be to use tretinoin or hydroxy acids on Monday, Wednesday, and Friday, then another topical product on the intervening days. Discuss this approach with your dermatologist. Once you find what works best for you, stick with it.

With that in mind, here's what to consider at various stages in your life.

Your Twenties

More than likely, you have no visible wrinkling. Lucky you! At this point (usually in your twenties and early thirties) wrinkles have not yet made their mark. The very best action you can take now is to get sunscreen savvy. Use sunscreens religiously.

Very important: Resist the urge to use tanning beds. It has been estimated that 15 to 30 minutes a day in a tanning booth is as skin damaging as a day in the sun.

Be sure to moisturize your skin once a day if it is dry.

Your Thirties

By your early to mid-thirties, you may begin to notice the development of fine lines, particularly when your face is animated. Barely perceptible wrinkles may begin showing up as crow's-feet, frown lines, or smile lines.

To put wrinkles on hold, use a sunscreen daily and moisturize your skin if it is dry. In addition, consider one of the following products in your skin-rejuvenation plan:

◊ Retin-A or Renova (often recommended for younger patients who want to forestall the aging effects of sun exposure)

◊ Alpha or beta hydroxy acids

◊ Topical antioxidants

◊ Topical coenzyme Q10

Your Forties and Fifties

By now, wrinkles may be obvious when your face is at rest, because of a combination of normal aging and time spent in the sun. In addition, skin has lost its natural glow and normal color. To prevent further damage, always wear sunscreen and moisturize if you need to.

Talk to your dermatologist about the following products and treatments:

◊ Retin-A or Renova

◊ Kinerase (if you're unable to tolerate Retin-A or Renova)

◊ Alpha or beta hydroxy acids

◊ Topical antioxidants

◊ Topical coenzyme Q10

◊ Marine products

◊ Superficial or medium-depth chemical peels

◊ Skin resurfacing

◊ Injections of botulinum toxin

◊ Dermal fillers

Here's something else to consider now: Hormone replacement therapy (HRT). HRT involves treatment with estrogen, often along with progestin (a synthetic version of the hormone progesterone). Estrogen is often recommended for preventing diseases such as osteoporosis and for generally maintaining good health beyond menopause.

After menopause, your skin begins to age more rapidly. Collagen decreases, and skin becomes drier and less elastic. These changes are associated with the natural decline in estrogen that occurs with menopause.

Some research suggests that both topical and oral estrogen therapy have antiaging effects on skin. Whereas tretinoin and hydroxy acids are excellent defenses against photoaging, estrogen appears to work powerfully against intrinsic aging. In fact, many skin specialists feel that it keeps skin taut, increases its thickness, and delays the development of wrinkles.

In a study conducted at the University of Vienna Medical School, women approaching menopause experienced improved skin elasticity and firmness, an increase in skin moisture, and a reduction in wrinkle depth after using top-

ical estrogen for six months. When researchers microscopically examined skin biopsies taken from the subjects, they
discovered that the number of collagen fibers had increased significantly. A similar study conducted in Finland
demonstrated that topical estrogen, applied once a day, increased the amount of skin collagen in postmenopausal
women after just three months of treatment.

There's more evidence supporting an antiaging benefit
of topical estrogen: French researchers tested the effects of
an estrogen cream (Premarin) on 54 postmenopausal
women, aged 52 to 70, who had moderate to severe signs
of facial aging. Each night, half of the group applied one
gram of the cream to their faces; the other half used a
placebo. In the morning, all of the women applied a sunscreen with an SPF of 15 to their faces. The experiment
lasted 24 weeks.

By the end of the experimental period, two fascinating
findings emerged. First, skin thickness increased more in
the Premarin-treated group than in the placebo group. Second, wrinkles improved significantly in those who used
Premarin. No side effects were reported either.

If these studies are any indication, it looks like topical
estrogen is a promising agent against intrinsic aging.

But so is oral estrogen, according to other research. In
one large-scale study, investigators analyzed the skin and
lifestyle habits (smoking and sun exposure) of 3,875 postmenopausal women, aged 40 and older. After adjusting for
sun exposure and smoking, the investigators discovered
that the estrogen-takers were less likely to have dry skin,
but more significantly, had fewer wrinkles than women
who were not on estrogen therapy.

The investigators drew the following conclusion:
"These results strongly suggest that estrogen use prevents
dry skin and wrinkling, thus extending the potential
benefits of postmenopausal estrogen therapy to include

protection against age-related menopause-associated dermatologic conditions."

There are two dermatologic inconveniences associated with taking oral estrogen, however. One is melasma, a condition in which large dark spots of increased pigmentation develop on skin. Fortunately, using a sunscreen can prevent it. For existing melasma, a prescription skin-bleaching agent such as hydroquinone works well.

The other skin-related side effect is acne. It is easily treated with an over-the-counter product containing benzoyl peroxide; oral antibiotics; or topical tretinoin. If the acne doesn't resolve in a few weeks, talk to your physician about discontinuing HRT or switching to a lower dosage or a different formulation.

Long-term HRT can increase the risk of breast cancer and is becoming a concern among women and physicians. If considering estrogen replacement therapy, you must weigh potential health risks and discuss them with your physician. At this stage in your life, the preservation of overall health may be more important than treating a cosmetic condition with estrogen.

Topical and oral estrogens are prescription drugs. A nonprescription topical hormone is Ethocyn, which has been shown in research to increase elastin in mature skin. Manufactured by Chantal Skin Care, Ethocyn is applied twice a day to areas of the skin most affected by aging. Although it can be used in conjunction with tretinoin or hydroxy acids, you should discuss pros and cons of combination therapy with your dermatologist.

Your Sixties and Beyond

At this stage in life, you may have deep, coarse wrinkling over your entire face, particularly if you have severe photodamage. Plus, your skin may appear yellowish gray in tone. According to skin experts, topical therapy such as tretinoin, hydroxy acids, antioxidants, or estrogen will still do your skin some favors. But to undo deep lines and restore skin integrity, it may be time to explore more aggressive cosmetic procedures such as:

◊ Deep chemical peels

◊ Skin resurfacing

◊ Face-lift

YOUR NEW LOOK

For some women, wrinkles just don't matter because they're comfortable with their looks and embrace the aging process. For others, wrinkles do matter because they want to look as youthful as they can, for as long as they can. Both attitudes are healthy.

If you're among those who choose to pursue a wrinkle-reduction program, the extra effort—and the benefits it brings—is well worth it, physically and emotionally. Just remember, though: Youthfulness is much more than just having a wrinkle-free complexion. It's a state of mind and spirit that never declines, even as time marches on.

References

A portion of the information in this book comes from medical journals; medical articles in both popular and scientific publications; books and booklets; promotional literature from skin-care companies; Internet sources; and computer searches of medical databases of research abstracts.

CHAPTER ONE
Your Amazing Skin

Bisacre, M., et al. 1984. *The illustrated encyclopedia of the human body.* New York: Exeter Books.

Elias, P. M. 1981. Epidermal lipids, membranes, and keratinization. *International Journal of Dermatology* 20: 1–19.

Kligman, A. M., and J. A. Graham. 1989. The psychology of appearance in the elderly. *Clinics in Geriatric Medicine* 5: 213–222.

West, M. D. 1994. The cellular and molecular biology of skin aging. *Archives of Dermatology* 130: 87–95.

CHAPTER TWO
How Your Face Ages

Bergfeld, W. G. 1999. A lifetime of healthy skin: implications for women. *International Journal of Fertility and Women's Medicine* 44: 83–95.

Burke, K. E. 1990. Facial wrinkles. Prevention and non-surgical correction. *Postgraduate Medicine* 88: 207–228.

Campisi, J. 1998. The role of cellular senescence in skin aging. *Journal of Investigative Dermatology* 3: 1–5.

Editor. 1997. Shape up your skin. *Ladies' Home Journal,* March, pp. 150–153.

Editor. 1991. Smoking's new wrinkle. *Prevention,* October, p. 12.

Glogau, R. 1997. Physiologic and structural changes associated with aging skin. *Dermatologic Clinics* 15: 555–559.

Hadshiew, I. M., et al. 2000. Skin aging and photoaging: the role of DNA damage and repair. *American Journal of Contact Dermatitis* 2: 19–25.

Hayflick, L. 1989. Antecedents of cell aging research. *Experimental Gerontology* 24: 355–365.

Kligman, A. M., et al. 1985. The anatomy and pathogenesis of wrinkles. *British Journal of Dermatology* 113: 37–42.

Kolb, S. 2000. Prevention and treatment of facial aging. On-line: www.ebody.com.

Lawrence, N. 2000. New and emerging treatments for photoaging. *Dermatologic Clinics* 18: 99–112.

National Women's Health Resource Center. 1996. Smoking ravages skin. *National Women's Health Report* 18: 7.

Pierard, G. E., et al. 1998. Ageing and rheological properties of facial skin in women. *Gerontology* 44: 159–161.

Sherris, D. A., et al. 1998. Comprehensive treatment of the

aging face—cutaneous and structural rejuvenation. *Mayo Clinic Proceedings* 73: 139–146.

West, M. D. 1994. The cellular and molecular biology of skin aging. *Archives of Dermatology* 130: 87–95.

Yaar, M., and B. A. Gilchrest. 1998. Aging versus photoaging: postulated mechanisms and effectors. *Journal of Investigative Dermatology* 3: 47–51.

Yin, L., et al. 2000. Alternations of extracellular matrix induced by tobacco smoke extract. *Archives of Dermatological Research* 292: 188–194.

CHAPTER THREE
First Things First: The New Sunscreens

Allen, J. E. 1993. Drug-induced photosensitivity. *Clinical Pharmacy* 12: 580–587.

Borowitz, S. M. 1998. Drug-induced photosensitivity. *Pediatric Pharmacotherapy.* On-line: www.medscape.com.

Boyer, P. 1994. Environmental protection for you skin. *Prevention,* September, pp. 120–122.

Burke, K. E. 1990. Facial wrinkles. Prevention and nonsurgical correction. *Postgraduate Medicine* 88: 207–228.

Cayrol, C., et al. 1999. A mineral sunscreen affords genomic protection against ultraviolet (UV) B and UVB radiation: in vitro and in situ assays. *British Journal of Dermatology* 141: 250–258.

Djerassi, D. 1997. The role of protective vitamins and sunscreens in the new, high-performance cosmetics. *Drug & Cosmetic Industry* 161: 52–56.

Editor. 2000. Safe in the sun. *Consumer Reports,* July, pp. 54–55.

Editor. 1998. Sun sensitivity. *Mayo Clinic Health Letter* 16:6.

Foley, D. 1987. How to live safely in the sun. *Prevention,* April, pp. 86–88, 122–125.

Freed, J. C. 1998. Saving your skin. *Town & Country,* July, pp. 88–94.

Gould, J. W., et al. 1995. Cutaneous photosensitivity diseases induced by exogenous agents. *Journal of the American Academy of Dermatology* 33: 551–573.

Griffiths, C. E. 1999. Drug treatment of photoaged skin. *Drugs & Aging* 14: 289–301.

Guttman, C. 1998. Zinc oxide, vitamin C products boost protection against UV rays. *Dermatology Times,* October, p. 11.

Katiyar, S. K., et al. 1999. Prevention of UVB-induced immunosuppression in mice by the green tea polyphenol (-)-epigallocatechin-3-gallate may be associated with alterations in IL-10 and IL-12 production. *Carcinogenesis* 20: 2117–2124.

Lawrence, N. 2000. New and emerging treatments for photoaging. *Dermatologic Clinics* 18: 99–112.

Lim, H. W., et al. 1990. Chronic actinic dermatitis. Study of the spectrum of chronic photosensitivity in 12 patients. *Archives of Dermatology* 126: 317–323.

Mathews-Roth, M. M. 1986. Systemic photoprotection. *Dermatologic Clinics* 4: 335–339.

Larson, D. E. 1990. *Mayo Clinic Family Healthbook.* New York: William Morrow and Company.

McLean, D. I., and R. Gallagher. 1998. Sunscreens. Use and misuse. *Dermatologic Clinics* 16: 219–226.

Mitchnick, M. A., et al. 1998. A review of sunscreen safety and efficacy. *Photochemistry and Photobiology* 68: 243–256.

Mitchnick, M. A., et al. 1999. Microfine zinc oxide (Z-Cote) as a photostable UVA/UVB sunblock agent. *Journal of the American Academy of Dermatology* 40: 85–90.

Reid, C. D. 1996. Chemical photosensitivity—another reason to be careful in the sun. *FDA Consumer.* May. Online: www.fda.gov.

Rhodes, L. E., and S. I. White. 1998. Dietary fish oil as a photoprotective agent in hydroa vacciniforme. *British Journal of Dermatology* 138: 173–178.

Wessel, H. 1998. Dermatologists praise new sunscreen ingredient. *Orlando Sentinel,* June 3, p. E3.

Wentzell, J. M. 1996. Sunscreens: an ounce of prevention. *American Family Physician* 53: 1713–1733.

CHAPTER FOUR
Youth-Enhancing Moisturizers

Boyer, P. 1988. Beauty basics for changing times. *Prevention,* January, pp. 56–58.

Broadhurst, C. L. 1999. More than skin deep. *Nutrition Science News,* November. On-line: www.healthwellexchange.com.

Editor. 2000. The skin game. *Consumer Reports,* January. On-line: www.consumerreport.com.

Jackson, E. M. 1992. Facial moisturizers and wrinkles. *Dermatologic Nursing* 4: 205–207.

Kligman, A. M., and A. M. Dattner. 1999. Toward optimum health: the experts respond to aging skin. *Journal of Women's Health & Gender-Based Medicine* 8: 1021–1025.

Lazar, A. P., and P. Lazar. Dry skin, water, and lubrication. *Dermatologic Clinics* 9: 45–51.

Loden, M., and M. Lindberg. 1991. The influence of a single application of different moisturizers on the skin capacitance. *Acta Dermato-Venereologica* 71: 79–82.

McCallion, R., and A. Li Wan Po. Dry and photo-aged skin: manifestations and management. *Journal of Clinical Pharmacy and Therapeutics* 18: 15–32.

Perricone, N. (ed.) 1998. Taking a closer look at xerosis in the elderly. *Skin & Aging* 6: 16–18.

Serup, J. 1992. A three-hour test for rapid comparison of

effects of moisturizers and active constituents (urea). *Acta Dermato-Venereologica* 177: 29–33.

Spencer, T. S. 1988. Dry skin and skin moisturizers. *Clinics in Dermatology* 6: 24–28.

Wehr, R. F., and L. Krochmal. 1987. Considerations for selecting a moisturizer. *Cutis* 39: 512–515.

CHAPTER FIVE
The Remarkable Retinoids

Bergfeld, W. G. 1999. A lifetime of healthy skin: implications for women. *International Journal of Fertility and Women's Medicine* 44: 83–95.

Duell, E. A., et al. 1997. Unoccluded retinol penetrates human skin in vivo more effectively than unoccluded retinyl palmitate or retinoic acid. *Journal of Investigative Dermatology* 109: 301–305.

Editor. 1996. Tretinoin (Renova) approved for treatment of wrinkles. *Medical Sciences Bulletin* 18: 2.

Editor. 2000. Renova. On-line: www.wrinklereport.com.

Fischer, J. 1996. The skinny on aging. *Newsday,* March 20, p. B15.

Fluhr, J. W. 1999. Tolerance profile of retinol, retinaldehyde and retinoic acid under maximized and long-term clinical conditions. *Dermatology* 199: 57–60.

Garrido, M. 1999. Understanding the uses, effects of retinol on skin. *The News,* November 17 (no page number provided).

Gilchrest, B. A. 1997. Treatment of photodamage with topical tretinoin: an overview. *Journal of the American Academy of Dermatology* 36: S27–S36.

Griffiths, C. E., et al. 1992. Mechanisms of action of retinoic acid in skin repair. *British Journal of Dermatology* 127: 21–24.

———. 1999. Drug treatment of photoaged skin. *Drugs & Aging* 14: 289–301.

Kang, S. 1995. Application of retinol to human skin in vivo induces epidermal hyperplasia and cellular retinoid binding proteins characteristic of retinoic acid but without measurable retinoic acid levels or irritation. *Journal of Investigative Dermatology* 105: 549–556.

Katsambas, A. D., and A. C. Katoulis. 1999. Topical retinoids in the treatment of aging of the skin. *Advances in Experimental Medicine and Biology* 455: 477–482.

Kligman, A. M. 1996. Topical retinoic acid (tretinoin) for photoaging: conceptions and misperceptions. *Cutis* 57: 142–144.

———. 1997. Topical treatments for photoaged skin. *Postgraduate Medicine* 102: 115–118, 123–126.

———. 1998. The growing importance of topical retinoids in clinical dermatology: a retrospective and prospective analysis. *Journal of the American Academy of Dermatology* 39: S2–S7.

Lister, P. 1990. Inspector skin. *American Health,* April, pp. 56–61.

Nidus Information Service. 1999. Skin wrinkles. On-line: www.well-connected.com.

Salagnac, V., et al. 1991. Treatment of actinic aging with topical vitamin A in different concentrations. *Revue Française de Gynécologie et d'Obstétrique* 86: 458–460.

Saurat, J. H. 1995. Retinoids and aging. *Hormone Research* 43: 89–92.

Silverstein, D. B. 1996. New wrinkles in skin cream. Renova: How does it stack up? *Newsday,* July 8, p. B13.

Toufexis, A. 1987. Antidote to all those wrinkles? *Time,* December 14, p. 90.

Varani, J., et al. 2000. Vitamin A antagonizes decreased cell growth and elevated collagen-degrading matrix metalloproteinases and stimulates collagen accumulation in naturally aged human skin. *Journal of Investigative Dermatology* 114: 480–486.

CHAPTER SIX
Skin-Smoothing Hydroxy Acids

Berardesca, E., et al. 1997. Alpha hydroxy acids modulate stratum corneum barrier function. *British Journal of Dermatology* 137: 934–938.

Bernstein, E. F., et al. 1997. Citric acid increases viable epidermal thickness and glycosaminoglycan content of sun-damaged skin. *Dermatologic Surgery* 23: 689–694.

Clark, C. P. 1996. Alpha hydroxy acids in skin care. *Clinics in Plastic Surgery* 23: 49–56.

Ditre, C. M., et al. 1996. Effects of alpha-hydroxy acids on photoaged skin: a pilot clinical, histologic, and ultrastructural study. *Journal of the American Academy of Dermatology* 34: 187–195.

Food and Drug Administration. 1999. Alpha hydroxy acids for skin care: smooth sailing or rough seas. *The FDA Consumer.* March/April. On-line: www.fda.gov.

Guttman, C. 1997. Benefits of alpha hydroxy acids finally supported by hard data. *Dermatology Times,* January 1, p. 46.

Jennings, L. 1999. Facing age. *Washington Times,* September 12, p. D4.

Kim, S. J., and Y. H. Won. 1998. The effect of glycolic acid on cultured human skin fibroblasts: cell proliferative effect and increased collagen synthesis. *Journal of Dermatology* 25: 85–89.

Kneedler, J. A., et al. 1998. Understanding alpha-hydroxy acids. *Dermatology Nursing* 10: 247–259.

Lawrence, N. 2000. New and emerging treatments for photoaging. *Dermatologic Clinics* 18: 99–112.

Perricone, N. V., and J. C. DiNardo. 1996. Photoprotective and antiinflammatory aspects of topical glycolic acid. *Dermatologic Surgery* 22: 435–437.

Sepp, D. T. 1998. The ABCs of alpha-hydroxy acids. *Les*

Nouvelles Esthetiques, December. On-line: www. shikai.com.

Smith, W. P. 1996. Epidermal and dermal effects of topical lactic acid. *Journal of the American Academy of Dermatology* 35: 388–391.

Stiller, M. J., et al. 1996. Topical 8% glycolic acid and 8% L-lactic acid creams for the treatment of photodamaged skin. A double-blind vehicle-controlled clinical trial. *Archives of Dermatology* 132: 631–636.

Vidt, D. G., and W. F. Bergfeld. 1997. Cosmetic use of alpha-hydroxy acids. *Cleveland Clinic Journal of Medicine* 64: 327–329.

Whitmore, S. E. 1997. Effects of alpha-hydroxy acids on photoaged skin. *Journal of the American Academy of Dermatology* 36: 654–655.

Wolfe, Y. L. 1997. Smooth away wrinkles: new way to revitalize older skin. *Prevention,* September, p. 47.

CHAPTER SEVEN
The Skin Antioxidants

Alster, T. S., and T. B. West. 1998. Effect of topical vitamin C on postoperative carbon dioxide laser resurfacing erythema. *Dermatologic Surgery* 24: 331–334.

Blatt, T., et al. 1999. Modulation of oxidative stress in human aging skin. *Zeitschrift für Gerontologie und Geriatrie* 32: 83–88.

Berneburg, M., et al. Singlet oxygen mediates the UVA-induced generation of the photoaging-associated mitochondrial common deletion. *Journal of Biological Chemistry* 274: 15345–15349.

Darr, D., et al. 1992. Topical vitamin C protects porcine skin from ultraviolet radiation-induced damage. *British Journal of Dermatology* 127: 247–253.

———. 1996. Effectiveness of antioxidants (vitamin C

and E) with and without sunscreens as topical photo-protectants. *Acta Dermato-Venereologica* 76: 264–268.

Dreher, F., et al. 1999. Effect of topical antioxidants on UV-induced erythema formation when administered after exposure. *Dermatology* 198: 52–55.

Fryer, M. J. 1993. Evidence for the photoprotective effects of vitamin E. *Photochemistry and Photobiology* 58: 304–312.

Gehring, W., et al. 1998. Influence of vitamin E acetate on stratum corneum hydration. *Arzneimittelforschung* 48: 772–775.

Greco, R. J. 2000. Topical vitamin C. *Plastic and Reconstructive Surgery* 105: 464–465.

Hoppe, K., et al. 1999. Coenzyme Q10, a cutaneous antioxidant and energizer. *Biofactors* 9: 371–378.

Keller, K. L., and N. A. Fenske. 1998. Use of vitamins A, C, and E and related compounds in dermatology. A review. *Journal of the American Academy of Dermatology* 39: 611–625.

Kohen, R. 1999. Skin antioxidants: their role in aging and in oxidative stress. New approaches for their evaluation. *Biomedicine and Pharmacotherapy* 53: 181–192.

Lee, J., et al. 2000. Carotenoid supplementation reduces erythema in human skin after simulated solar radiation exposure. *Proceedings of the Society for Experimental Biology and Medicine* 223: 170–174.

Martell, C. 2000. A new wrinkle in skin care. *Wisconsin State Journal,* March 5. On-line: www.cellex-c.com.

Nachbar, F., and H. C. Korting. 1995. The role of vitamin E in normal and damaged skin. *Journal of Molecular Medicine* 73: 7–17.

Pehr, K., and R. R. Forsey. 1993. Why don't we use vitamin E in dermatology? *Canadian Medical Association Journal* 149: 1247–1253.

Perricone, N. V. 2000. Research and clinical documentation. The use of topical ascorbyl palmitate and alpha lipoic acid for aging skin. On-line: www.nvperri-conemd.com.

Podda, M., et al. 1996. Kinetic study of cutaneous and sub-cutaneous distribution following topical application of [7,8-14C]rac-alpha-lipoic acid onto hairless mice. *Biochemical Pharmacology* 23: 627–633.

ProCyte Corporation. 2000. Product information. On-line: www.procyte.com.

Pugliese, P. T. 1998. The skin's antioxidant systems. *Dermatology Nursing* 10: 401–416.

Rampoldi, R., et al. 1990. Topical vitamin E and ultraviolet radiation on human skin. *Medicina Cutanea Ibero-Latino-Americana* 18: 269–272.

Ricciarelli, R., et al. 1999. Age-dependent increase of collagenase expression can be reduced by alpha-tocopherol via protein kinase C inhibition. *Free Radical Biology and Medicine* 27: 729–737.

Tanaka, H., et al. 1993. The effect of reactive species on the biosynthesis of collagen and glycosaminoglycans in cultured human dermal fibroblasts. *Archives of Dermatological Research* 285: 352–355.

Traikovich, S. S. 1999. Use of topical ascorbic acid and its effects on photodamaged skin topography. *Archives of Otolaryngology—Head and Neck Surgery* 125: 1091–1098.

Stahl, W., et al. 2000. Carotenoids and carotenoids plus vitamin E protect against ultraviolet light-induced erthema in humans. *American Journal of Clinical Nutrition* 71: 795–798.

Steenvoorden, D., and G. van Henegouwen. 1997. The use endogenous antioxidants to improve photoprotection. *Journal of Photochemistry and Photobiology* 41: 1–10.

CHAPTER EIGHT
Return-to-Youth Botanicals

Calabrese, V., et al. 1999. Oxidative stress and antioxidants at skin biosurface: a novel antioxidant from lemon oil capable of inhibiting oxidative damage to the skin. *Drugs Under Experimental and Clinical Research* 25: 281–287.

Cossins, E., et al. 1998. ESR studies of vitamin C generation, order of reactivity of natural source phytochemical preparations. *Biochemistry and Molecular Biology International* 45: 583–597.

Duke, J. A. 1997. *The green pharmacy*. Emmaus, PA: Rodale Press.

Fields, K. A. 2000. Skin breakthroughs in the year 2000. *International Journal of Fertility and Women's Medicine* 45: 175–181.

Gabor, L. 1992. Beautify with botanicals. *Prevention*, September, pp. 124–127.

Goldemberg, R. 1998. Natural ingredients. Drug & Cosmetic Industry, February. On-line: www.findarticles.com.

Hunt, P. 1999. Looking good. *Vegetarian Times,* September. On-line: www.findarticles.com.

Ichihashi, M., et al. 2000. Preventive effect of antioxidant on ultraviolet-induced skin cancer in mice. *Journal of Dermatological Science* 23 Supplement 1: S45–S50.

Kligman, A. M., and A. M. Dattner. 1999. Toward optimum health: the experts respond to aging skin. *Journal of Women's Health & Gender-Based Medicine* 8: 1021–1025.

Lowe, B. 2000. Indian influence. *Nutritional Outlook* 3: 31–39.

Madley, R. H. 2000. Going beneath the surface in anti-aging skin care. *Nutraceuticals World* 3: 82–86.

Saliou, C., et al. Antioxidants modulate acute solar ultraviolet radiation-induced NF-kappa-B activation in human kerintocyte cell line. *Free Radical Biology and Medicine* 26: 174–183.

Tixier, J. M., et al. 1984. Evidence by in vivo and in vitro studies that binding of pycnogenols to elastin affects its rate of degradation by elastases. *Biochemical Pharmacology* 33: 3933–3939.

Virgili, F., et al. 1998. Procyanidins extracted from pine bark protect alpha-tocopherol in ECV 304 endothelial cells challenged by activated RAW 264,7 macrophages: role of nitric oxide and peroxynitrite. *FEBS Letters* 431: 315–318.

Zink, W. 1996. Pycnogenol and skincare. *Drug & Cosmetic Industry News* 158: 44–47.

CHAPTER NINE
Young Skin Secrets from the Sea

Ahava. 2000. Product information. On-line: www.ahava.com.

Aurora Group. 2000. Vivida product information. On-line: www.theauroragroup.com.

Bionax. 2000. Imedeen product information. On-line: www.bionax.com.

Booth, C. 2000. Crème de la mer. The cream created by a NASA rocket scientist. On-line: www.time.com.

Carpio-Obesco, M. P., et al. 1999. Desert ecosystems: similarities, characteristics, and health benefits. *Reviews on Environmental Health* 14: 257–267.

Coleman, C. 1998. More than skin deep. *Soap Perfumery & Cosmetics* 71: 37.

Eskelinen, A., and J. Santalahti. 1992. Special natural cartilage polysaccharides for the treatment of sun-damaged skin in females. *International Journal of Medical Research* 20: 99–105.

Estée Lauder Companies Inc. 2000. La mer. On-line: www.elcompanies.com.

Goldemberg, R. L. 1995. From the sea. *Drug & Cosmetic Industry* 157: 56–59.

————. 1997. Israeli cosmetics. *Drug & Cosmetic Industry* 160: 69–71.

Kieffer, M. E., and J. Efsen. 1998. Imedeen in the treatment of photoaged skin: an efficacy and safety trial over 12 months. *Journal of the European Academy of Dermatology and Venereology* 11: 129–136.

Lassus, A., et al. 1991. Imedeen for the treatment of degenerated skin in females. *Journal of International Medical Research* 19: 147–152.

————. 1992. The effect of Vivida cream as compared with placebo cream in the treatment of sun-damaged or age-damaged facial skin. *Journal of International Medical Research* 20: 381–391.

Heule, F. An oral approach to the treatment of photodamaged skin: a pilot study. *Journal of International Medical Research* 20: 273–278.

Ma'or, Z., et al. 1996. Dead Sea mineral-based cosmetics—facts and illusions. *Israel Journal of Medical Sciences* 32: S28–S35.

Rosenthal, M. L. 1964. Biological role and practice uses of squalene and squalane. In: *Cosmetics and the skin.* New York, NY: Reinhold Publishing Corp. On-line: www.earthportals.com.

CHAPTER TEN
Skin-Deep Beauty: Chemical Peels

American Academy of Dermatologists. 1999. Youthful skin made possible with advanced chemical peels and wrinkle fillers. October 27. Press release.

American Society of Plastic Surgeons. 1997. Chemical peel. On-line: www.plasticsurgery.org.

American Society of Plastic Surgeons. 1997. Skin rejuvenation. On-line: www.plasticsurgery.org.

Becker, F. F., et al. 1996. A histological comparison of 50% and 70% glycolic acid peels using solutions with various pHs. *Dermatologic Surgery* 22: 463–465.

Collawn, S. S., et al. 1998. Ultrastructural study of the skin after facial chemical peels and the effect of moisturization on wound healing. *Plastic and Reconstructive Surgery* 101: 1374–1379.

Dailey, R. A., et al. 1998. Histopathologic changes of the eyelid skin following trichloroacetic acid chemical peel. *Ophthalmic Plastic and Reconstructive Surgery* 14: 9–12.

Giese, S. Y., et al. 1997. The effect of chemosurgical peels and dermabrasion on dermal elastic tissue. *Plastic and Reconstructive Surgery* 100: 489–98.

Kligman, D., and A. M. Kligman. 1998. Salicylic acid peels for the treatment of photoaging. *Dermatologic Surgery* 24: 325–328.

Kneedler, J. A., et al. 1998. Understanding alpha-hydroxy acids. *Dermatology Nursing* 10: 247–259.

Matarasso, S. L., and R. G. Glogau. 1991. Chemical face peels. *Dermatologic Clinics* 9: 131–150.

Piacquadio, D., et al. 1996. Short contact 70% glycolic acid peels as a treatment for photodamaged skin. A pilot study. *Dermatologic Surgery* 22: 449–452.

Tse, Y., et al. 1996. A clinical and histologic evaluation of two medium-depth peels. Glycolic acid versus Jessner's trichloroacetic acid. *Dermatologic Surgery* 22: 781–786.

CHAPTER ELEVEN
Wrinkle Fillers

American Academy of Dermatology. 2000. Botulinum in the new millennium. August 3. Press release.

American Society of Plastic Surgeons. 2000. Injectable fillers in plastic surgery. On-line: www.plasticsurgery.org.

Caruthers, A., and J. Carruthers. 1998. History of the cosmetic use of botulinum A exotoxin. *Dermatologic Surgery* 24: 1168–1170.

Collagenesis. 2000. Dermalogen. On-line: www.collagenesis.

Devore, D. P., et al. 1994. Effectiveness of injectable filler materials for smoothing wrinkle lines and depressed scars. *Medical Progress Through Technology* 20: 243–250.

Editor. 2000. Plastic surgery. On-line: www.ebody.com.

Editor. 1987. Treatment of depressed cutaneous scars with gelatin matrix implant: a multicenter study. *Journal of the American Academy of Dermatology* 16: 1155–1162.

Food and Drug Administration. 1991. Collagen and liquid silicone injections. August. On-line: www.fda.gov.

Gold, M. H. 1994. The Fibril mechanism of action. A preliminary report. *Journal of Dermatologic Surgery and Oncology* 20: 586–590.

Guttman, C. 1999. New materials tested for soft tissue augmentation. *Dermatology Times,* February. On-line: www.findarticles.com.

Loftus, J. M. 2000. Collagen for filling wrinkles. On-line: www.drloftus.com.

Spira, M., and T. Rosen. 1993. Injectable soft tissue substitutes. *Clinics in Plastic Surgery* 20: 181–188.

Streit, M., et al. 1999. Soft tissue augmentation for treatment of wrinkles and scars of the face. *Therapeutische Umschau* 56: 212–218.

CHAPTER TWELVE
Antiaging Breakthroughs: Skin Resurfacing

American Academy of Dermatologists. 1999. New peeling technique offers lunchtime solution to skin resurfacing. March 20. Press release.

————. 2000. Electrosurgical resurfacing: a new option in facial rejuvenation. March 10. Press release.

————. 2000. New cosmetic procedures offer simple solutions to aging skin. August 3. Press release.

American Society of Plastic Surgeons. 2000. Dermabrasion and dermaplaning refinishing the skin. On-line: www.plasticsurgery.org.

————. 2000. Lasers in plastic surgery. On-line: www.plasticsurgery.org.

Boschert, S. 1999. Electrosurgical resurfacing seems safe so far. *Skin & Allergy News* 30: 29.

Burns, R. L., et al. 1999. Electrosurgical skin resurfacing: a new bipolar instrument. *Dermatologic Surgery* 25: 582–586.

Davis, J. 2000. Beyond lasers: pulse-light therapy for that fantasy face. July 27. On-line: www.webmd.com.

Editor. 2000. Plastic surgery. On-line: www.ebody.com.

Farrior, R. T. 1985. Dermabrasion in facial surgery. *Laryngoscope* 95: 534–545.

Hannapel, C. E. 1999. Non-ablative lasers can treat wrinkles. *Dermatology Times,* November. On-line: www.findarticles.com.

Lim, J. 1997. Carbon dioxide laser skin resurfacing. *NSC Bulletin.* On-line: www.nsc.gov.sg/bulletin.

Mooney, L. 2000. Reduce laser redness. *Prevention,* August, pp.104–105.

Nidus Information Service. 1999. Skin wrinkles. On-line: www.well-connected.com.

Stevens, J. 2000. Spotlight on cosmetic procedures: facing the future. *San Jose Mercury News,* August 13. On-line: www.svmagazine.com.

Weinstein, C., and M. Scheflan. 2000. Simultaneously combined ER:YAG and carbon dioxide laser (derma K) for skin resurfacing. *Clinics in Plastic Surgery* 27: 273–285.

CHAPTER THIRTEEN
The Age-Stopping Face-lift

American Society of Plastic & Reconstructive Surgeons. 2000. 1999 plastic surgery procedural statistics. On-line: www.plasticsurgery.org.
————. 2000. 1999 average surgeon's fees. On-line: www.plasticsurgery.org.
————. 2000. Blepharosplasty. On-line: www.plastic-surgery.org.
————. 2000. Facelift. On-line: www.plasticsurgery.org.
————. 2000. Forehead lift. On-line: www.plastic-surgery.org.
Landis, B. J. 1994. Facial cosmetic surgery: a primary care perspective. *The Nurse Practitioner* 19: 71–76.
Warmuth, I. P., et al. Dermatologic surgery into the next millennium: Part I. *Cutis* 64: 245–248.

CHAPTER FOURTEEN
Wrinkle-Reducing Makeup

American Society of Plastic and Surgeons. 2000. Camou-flage cosmetics. On-line: www.plasticsurgery.org.
Draelos, Z. D. 1996. Camouflaging techniques. *Cutis* 52: 362–364.
————. 1996. Camouflaging techniques and dermatologic surgery. *Dermatologic Surgery* 22: 1023–1027.
Editor. 1996. Beautiful skin. *Good Housekeeping,* January, p. 51.
Editor. 1996. The big cover-up. *Ladies' Home Journal,* April, pp. 54–55.
Editor. 2000. Faking it. *Ladies' Home Journal,* August, p. 22.
Editor. 1997. Look 5 years younger in 10 minutes. *Prevention,* July, p. 43.

Editor. 1991. Skin-perfecting makeup. *Ladies' Home Journal,* September, p. 29.

Editor. 1996. Your makeup at 30, 40, 50 and beyond. *Good Housekeeping,* October, p. 50.

Editor. 1995. Yours truly. *Weight Watchers Magazine,* October, p. 34.

Gaudoin, T. 1992. Makeup. *Harper's Bazaar,* September, p. 324.

Goldstein, M. M. 2000. The right foundation. *Town & Country,* August, p. 58.

Gooden, Charmaine. 1994. Be your own makeup artist. *Chatelaine,* June, p. 46.

Kligman, A. M., and J. A. Graham. 1989. The psychology of appearance in the elderly. *Clinics in Geriatric Medicine* 5: 213–222.

Meltzer-McGrath, M. 2000. Beauty know it all. *In Style,* February, p. 189.

Nidus Information Service. 1999. Skin wrinkles. On-line: www.well-connected.com.

Ogden-West, N. 1999. Cosmetics for the eye area after cosmetic procedures. *Skin Pharmacology and Applied Skin Physiology* 12: 120–124.

Rayner, V. L. 1995. Camouflage therapy. *Dermatologic Clinics* 13: 467–472.

Westmore, M. G. 1991. Makeup as an adjunct and aid to the practice of dermatology. *Dermatologic Clinics* 9: 81–88.

CHAPTER FIFTEEN
Your Personal Skin-Rejuvenation Program

American Academy of Dermatology. 2000. Skin stats. On-line: www.aad.org.

———. 2000. Topical management options for photodamaged skin. On-line: www.aad.org.

American Society of Plastic Surgeons (ck). 2000. Skin management. On-line: www.plasticsurgery.org.

Bilkis, M. R., and K. A. Mark. 1998. Mind-body medicine. Practical applications in dermatology. *Archives of Dermatology* 134: 1437–1441.

Bottone, E. J., et al. 1994. Loofah sponges as reservoirs and vehicles in the transmission of potentially pathogenic bacterial species to human skin. *Journal of Clinical Microbiology* 32: 469–472.

Boyer, P., and T. Walsh. 1997. Can hormone therapy save your skin? *Prevention,* July, pp. 121–123.

Boyer, P. 1985. How to keep your face "wash and wearable." *Prevention,* February, pp. 52–53.

———. 1997. One week to luminous skin. *Prevention,* April, pp. 73–75.

Creidi, P., et al. 1994. Effect of a conjugated oestrogen (Premarin) cream on aging facial skin. A comparative study with a placebo cream. *Maturitas* 19: 211–223.

Dunn, L. B., et al. 1997. Does estrogen prevent skin aging? Results from the first National Health and Nutrition Examination Survey. *Archives of Dermatology* 133: 339–342.

Editor. 2000. Raise a glass to better skin. *Prevention,* September, p. 138.

Glogau, R. 1997. Physiologic and structural changes associated with aging skin. *Dermatologic Clinics* 15: 555–559.

Kligman, A. M., and A. M. Dattner. 1999. Toward optimum health: the experts respond to aging skin, interview by Jodi Godfrey Meisler. *Journal of Women's Health & Gender-Based Medicine* 8: 1021–1025.

Morse, P. F., et al. 1989. Meta-analysis of placebo-controlled studies of the efficacy of Epogram in the treatment of atopic eczema. Relationship between plasma essential fatty acid changes and clinical response. *British Journal of Dermatology* 121: 75–90.

Nidus Information Service. 1999. Skin wrinkles. On-line: www.well-connected.com.

Schmidt, J. B., et al. 1996. Treatment of aging skin with topical estrogens. *International Journal of Dermatology* 35: 669–674.

Varila, E., et al. 1995. The effect of topical oestradiol on skin collagen of postmenopausal women. *British Journal of Obstetrics and Gynaecology* 102: 985–989.

About the Author

M aggie Greenwood-Robinson, Ph.D., is one of the country's top health and medical authors. She is the author of *The Bone Density Test, Hair Savers for Women: A Complete Guide to Preventing and Treating Hair Loss, The Cellulite Breakthrough, Natural Weight Loss Miracles, Kava Kava: The Ultimate Guide to Nature's Anti-Stress Herb,* and *21 Days to Better Fitness.* Plus, she is the coauthor of nine other fitness books, including the national bestseller *Lean Bodies, Lean Bodies Total Fitness, High Performance Nutrition, Power Eating,* and *50 Workout Secrets.*

Her articles have appeared in *Let's Live, Physical, Great Life, Shape* magazine, *Christian Single Magazine, Women's Sports and Fitness, Working Woman,* and many other publications. She is a member of the advisory board of *Physical* magazine. In addition, she has a doctorate in nutritional counseling, and is a certified nutritional consultant.